FINDING HOPE

My Journey Through Anorexia Nervosa Recovery

Jade Kidger

To my wonderful family and each and every single person who has supported me through my illness and recovery. I couldn't have done any of this without you.

PREFACE

Hello friends, whether you picked this book up because you're in need of reassurance and comfort, or just because you were interested, I can't tell you how thankful I am. I hope that everyone who reads this is healthy and happy and knows that they are loved, but realistically, I know that won't be the case. So to anyone who needs to hear this today, tomorrow, or anytime in the future, you are enough. You are loved, you are needed, and you are amazing.

Eating disorders are horrific. They are mean, they are ugly, and they destroy lives. Nobody chooses to have an eating disorder, and nobody deserves to have an eating disorder. Did you hear that? For those of you stuck in this tortuous battle - in case you were in any doubt, in case you needed somebody to say it for you, you do not deserve to have this illness. And if suffering from the illness wasn't enough, recovery is a constant fight. It is an everlasting battle between the easy choice and the brave choice, doing what your mind is telling you to do, or having the strength and the courage to do the opposite.

Throughout my journey I've met a huge number of people with eating disorders, and I truly believe that many of them are the strongest people I've ever met. I know that if I said that to their face they would simply laugh at me – it doesn't feel strong to sit at the dining table sobbing hysterically into a glass of milk, it doesn't feel strong to panic and begin to hyperventilate when a yoghurt is placed in front of you. But when your own mind is determined to torture you and break you down to nothing, just being brave enough to carry on is extraordinarily strong.

I debated for a long time whether to write about my journey or not. One of the awful aspects of eating disorders is the comparison between sufferers. My mind was always telling me that I must be the sickest, that I must eat less than everyone else, that I had to weigh the least and be the skinniest. I used to read all the time on the internet how much people ate at their sickest, and as soon as someone ate less than me I felt completely invalidated. I felt like I wasn't worthy of treatment because there were people out there that had it worse. So I've tried to avoid making anybody feel like this while they're reading about my experiences, I've tried to keep the numbers and the really specific, personal details of my illness to myself. I also think this is important because eating disorders are mental illnesses. It doesn't matter what my lowest weight was, or the number of calories that I ate on my worst day, because those things don't tell you what was going on in my mind. Nevertheless, if you are suffering yourself there will probably be bits that make your eating disorder perk up and want to compare.

So I tell you this – you are valid and your illness is valid, no matter what your lowest weight was, if you were ever underweight at all; no matter what you ate on your worst day; no matter how many times you were hospitalised, if you were hospitalised at all; or how much medication you're on. You are valid if you've been suffering for a day, or for a month, or for a year. You are valid if you have experienced all of the same struggles I had, or whether your struggles are entirely different. You are totally and wholly valid no matter the circumstances of your illness, and you deserve treatment regardless of how you compare yourself to others.

In the end I decided that it's important for me to make sense of everything that I've been through by writing about it. I think the process of writing has allowed me to discover more about my eating disorder than I would ever have done otherwise. It has allowed my family to better understand what I've been through, and it's given me the chance to say things to them that I could never have said out loud. Writing for me has been extremely therapeutic and I hope that people reading my book will find it as helpful as I have found creating it.

For the purposes of this book I've called myself Jade. That isn't my real name, but I'm not sure I'm ready to fully open myself up to the world yet. I know that seems stupid, as I'm about to share some of the deepest and most intimate details of my life with you, but for some reason by writing under a pen name, I feel more confident. I feel like I can share my most precious secrets. Everything else apart from my name is completely true. Every feeling, every thought that I describe, however horrible and however unpleasant, are exactly what I went through during my illness and recovery.

Although I'm trying to remain relatively anonymous, and although I'm not sure I'm comfortable sharing my name, here is a little bit about me: I'm a medical student in the UK, however I had almost 2 years away from medical school to focus on anorexia recovery. This wasn't by choice, but I know now that it was best for me.

I've had a lot of ups and downs, and sometimes it's felt like I've gotten worse before I got better, but even though my progress has been relatively slow, it has still been progress. There's no timeline for recovery; for some people it takes a month, and for some people it takes years.

This book is my little project which has helped me so much to understand myself. It contains my thoughts, my feelings, and whatever else goes on in the deepest, darkest corners of my mind. It contains the good, the bad, the ugly, and most importantly, the truth. A couple of years ago I would have never believed I'd be in a position to be so open about my struggles with mental health, but now I'm sharing my journey with you. This book was not written as a guide to recovery, and I'm aware that some of the contents might be hard to read. But it is my story, and I hope it can provide some level of comfort or understanding to those most in need.

ME

Before I begin talking about my eating disorder, I want to talk a bit about me. Despite this book mainly focussing on my experiences with anorexia, I'm still a human being - there are so many other sides to me than my eating disorder.

I've always been happy. As a child I was outgoing, funny, and so chatty that I'm sure even my parents prayed for me to stop talking at times. School was good, family life was good, there really wasn't anything in my life that I can see as a trigger for my mental health battle. I grew up with two extremely loving parents, and an older sister and younger brother who I got on incredibly well with. Of course there was the odd disagreement, but underneath that we all loved each other.

I always worked hard. In school, in my hobbies,

I always put in the maximum amount of effort. I got brilliant grades and I knew that my future was bright. At the age of eighteen I achieved top grades in my A Levels and went off to medical school to become a doctor. It was everything I wanted and more. I was thriving off my new-found independence and becoming a proper, respectable adult. I always imagined that I would be a forensic pathologist when I qualified (a doctor who performs autopsies and determines how someone has died) but medical school opened up a huge array of possibilities, and I was unbelievably excited to explore them.

Then my life changed. Not all at once, but little by little anorexia began to creep up on me. Of course, I didn't recognise it for what it was at first; I guess if I had then my recovery might have been that little bit quicker and easier. Subtle changes began to occur – I wanted to become healthier, I wanted to become fitter. I honestly don't believe those little changes were signs of an eating disorder when they began, but somehow everything spiralled and my mind became a very dark place.

Once the illness took a proper hold of me it worsened so quickly and so viciously that there wasn't time to process what was happening. It took hold of me so strongly that it felt impossible to pull myself out of its clutches. I was still away at university, just twenty years old, struggling alone and scared.

I'm going to talk a lot in this book about how awful having an eating disorder is, but looking back there must have been some element that I secretly enjoyed, which kept the monster alive inside of me. I think that it made me feel strong, it made me feel powerful, like I was achieving something amazing. I was resisting temptation. However the illness is toxic. There were so many more bad moments than good, and the anxiety that developed inside of me was almost paralysing.

I'm also going to talk about how brave it is and how strong it is to recover from anorexia. However I want you to know that in the moment it feels anything but brave and strong. It feels like you're weak, like you're giving in to temptation. Looking back I can acknowledge how courageous I was, but at the time I felt like I was losing a battle every time I put a morsel of food in my mouth.

But this is just one account of someone with an eating disorder. Unfortunately there are so many more people out there who have suffered differently to me, who have suffered worse than me. This is my story.

'In the beginning there was only
fear. But she took it, and from it
she crafted her weapons – weapons
which would make her unstoppable.'

MY STORY

I t all started out so innocently. I just wanted to be a bit healthier, I just wanted to feel good about myself. But it spiralled into paralysing fear. Fear of gaining weight, fear of losing control, fear of becoming 'unhealthy'.

My whole life quickly became dominated by calories. The number of calories in an apple or a carrot or a piece of broccoli. I was addicted to looking at nutrition labels; I was a human encyclopaedia on the calorie content of different fruits. I set myself limits on how many calories I was allowed to consume in a day, and every day I would strive to lower the limit. I saw it as a challenge, and I succeeded every time. I felt good about myself. My mind felt so strong, so powerful, even though my body was becoming weaker by the day.

My kitchen scales became my best friend. While

everyone else was out at the pub or enjoying a pizza, I would be left at home weighing out my strawberries to the exact gram. Eating more than a certain number of calories was unacceptable, eating more than the recommended serving size was not allowed.

And then came the exercise: running my body right up to complete exhaustion. Hating every second of it but feeling so much worse when I didn't do it. Feeling lazy and disgusting when I lay in bed instead of getting up and working out, even though I'd done so much the day before. The voice in my head wouldn't let me rest – I had to earn my food. I had to earn my right to eat. And the purging. Trying to vomit to rid myself of the calories and sobbing into the toilet when I couldn't quite manage it. I was a freak, I was so ashamed.

The hunger consumed me. Every single minute of every single day, my body screamed out for food. It ripped through me, the constant ache of my stomach pleading with me to eat. It permeated my insides, my hollow, empty insides. It would crescendo to the point where I didn't think I could stand it anymore – it tortured me, it tore me apart from the inside out. Yet still my mind forbade me to eat, still my mind was intent on starving me.

I deteriorated extremely quickly, but those few

months felt like the longest months of my life. I was living day by day, hour by hour, struggling through each minute until I was 'allowed' to eat again. I hit rock bottom, I sunk further than I ever thought possible, I broke into a million tiny pieces. I tried pulling myself together – I thought that it would be easy to stop this insane addiction, I thought that it would be simple, but I never succeeded. I was reluctant to get proper help because I felt like a fraud. This hadn't been going on long enough, I wasn't underweight enough, I wasn't worthy of help.

Despite all of the pain, despite all of the suffering, I never believed I was truly ill. The voice in my head, the voice telling me to do all of these crazy things told me that I didn't really have anorexia, that my whole illness was a lie. When I finally did seek help I didn't believe I had 'proper' anorexia. Even when I started seeing the psychiatrist, I didn't have 'proper' anorexia. I wasn't even ill enough when I was in hospital. There was always someone who had suffered longer than me, who had a lower BMI than me, and they were the real sufferers, not me. I was an intruder, pretending to be part of their inside circle when I really didn't belong.

But the truth is, there is no 'proper' way to have anorexia. Every time the voice told me that I wasn't ill enough, or managed to convince me that it didn't exist, it was a sign that my illness was becoming stronger, becoming more a part of my life. It told me that I was making everything up, I was faking the eating disorder, I was just doing it for attention; and I believed it. I believed it was my best friend, my biggest confidant, my unwavering companion.

It's these thoughts that make anorexia so dangerous. I'm not stupid. I look at my weight, at my body, at my diet, and I can see that I'm ill. But I don't feel it, and that voice inside my head telling me that I'm not ill is so much easier to listen to than the numbers and figures. Deep down inside I know I'm worth so much more than this, but the voice tells me otherwise. The voice screams the opposite, and I trust every word.

When I was first diagnosed I felt like my freedom had been viciously ripped away from me: I couldn't drive, I couldn't exercise, I couldn't even leave the house by myself due to my body being so weak and damaged. But I hadn't been truly free for a long time. I'd been trapped by a horrible, unrelenting force slowly stripping me of my dignity and pride. I'd already been living on the dark side, recovery was my chance to see the light again.

THE DARKEST DAYS

I can't pinpoint which specific day was my darkest. Was it when I felt so sick and frail that I couldn't get out of bed? Was it the day that I cried for hours in the darkness of my bedroom, feeling too broken and too depressed to carry on? Or was it when I was simply too tired to fight, and I thought that the only way forward was to give up? Here's something I learnt about dark days: they will always come to an end, and you will always be able to try again tomorrow, or the day after, or whenever you feel ready. Because the universe is forgiving. The universe will always give you a second chance, because even though it might not feel like it a lot of the time, it has a wonderful plan for you. You just have to find enough courage within yourself to trust in the unknown to make it happen.

The darkest time in my life occurred when I should have been the happiest. Life is like that sometimes: the more potential you have to be happy, the more it will rip away from you. I was where I'd been aiming to get to for a long time – I was in my third year of medical school: finally starting my clinical placements, finally starting to feel somewhat like a doctor. It was hard – long days, difficult patients, endless studying; but it was bliss. It was the life I'd dreamed of for so long. I was honoured to walk onto the ward every morning and greet the nurses with a smile, but that smile was hiding a world of pain. I felt so incredibly lucky to be able to wear my uniform, but that uniform covered up a weak and failing body. So where did it all go wrong? How did my life go from fresh-faced doctor to pitiful patient in just a couple of months? Why was I chosen to suffer, instead of flourish and thrive like I should have been doing?

Perhaps it was because as a medical student, I was so hyperaware of what a bad diet can do to your body. Or maybe it was because I wanted to feel more in control of my life. Was it simply because I wanted to be more responsible for my health and it all got out of hand? Or was it because I longed to be the best at something, and being the thinnest was my way of achieving that?

I try to make sense of it all, I try to rationalise my thoughts and feelings and find a reason why everything happened, but in reality I was just ill. Just like some people catch a cold, just like some people get chicken pox or have a heart attack, I simply had an illness. It was nobody's fault, least of all mine, and there was no one to blame. There was no real explanation for why this happened to me, why the world decided to put me through everything that I went through. It was just fate I guess. Many millions of stars aligning at just the right time to set something massive into motion. I could spend days, weeks, agonising over why I was chosen to carry this burden. I could shout until my voice went hoarse that it wasn't fair, that I didn't deserve any of this. But what's the point? It's happened, and although we don't have the power to go back and change the past, we are in charge of our future. We have the freedom to choose what to do next: sink or swim, fight or flight, battle the monster or let it take your life.

Before my nightmare began I was taught at medical school about mental illness. I was taught how common it was for student doctors to suffer with mental illnesses, and where to go for help and support should my mental health ever deteriorate; but I always thought that those lessons didn't apply to me, I always presumed I was safe. Safe from the evil that affected other people's minds, messed with other people's lives. If someone would have told me that I would one day have to take time away from medical school because of my mental health, I wouldn't have believed them for a single second. If someone would have told me that a couple of years after starting university I would end up in hospital because of my mental health, I would have called them crazy. Things like that didn't happen to me: I was strong, I would never *let* anything like that happen to me.

But having a mental illness doesn't make you weak, just like having cancer or asthma doesn't make people weak. Mental illness isn't a choice: people don't choose to be depressed or anxious, they don't choose to have panic attacks or OCD. We don't choose to suffer, we don't choose to go through mental torture every single day, but we can choose to fight. We can choose to be warriors and battle for freedom. We can choose to be brave and courageous and fight for a life without mental illness. And most importantly we can choose to be kind. Kind to each other and kind to ourselves when things aren't going our way. Kind to our bodies and kind to our minds when they are being put through hell. Kind to those who couldn't get out of bed and to those who felt like giving up today. We are all just bruised and broken people fighting for our lives, fighting against a force that tries to convince us that we aren't worthy enough to eat and be loved. Trying to convince us that by starving ourselves, we will become better people, that we will become more worthy of love and affection.

People who suffer from mental illnesses aren't weak, we are some of the bravest and strongest people on Earth. We battle with our minds every single day, and yet we carry on. We carry on when all we want is to surrender. We carry on when our minds are telling us that we can't. We carry on when we are exhausted and can't take another step. We carry on until the end because we are soldiers; we are fighting with the hope that tomorrow will be a tiny bit better than today.

The darkest days of my eating disorder are reminiscent of dark days that I've managed to survive before. I can recall a period of time while I was studying for my A-levels where my mind told me some horrendous things: life was pointless, there was no hope, I may as well end my life because I had nothing to look forward to. My mind tried to convince me that I didn't deserve to live. My mind tried to convince me that I would be better off if I took my own life. My mind terrified me, yet I never divulged to anyone what was going on, and somehow the abhorrent thoughts eventually came to an end. It's only now that I look back and recognise how dangerous and how serious these thoughts were. Were they a premonition of what was to come, of what would befall me a couple of years later? But I didn't let it win that time, and I won't let it win this time either. This time I did the bravest thing and I asked for help. This time I knew I couldn't fight alone, and I reached out for support. Not at first, first I went through some dreadful and horrifying days, days that tortured me until I was too exhausted to stand, days that I thought would never come to an end. But finally I stood up and I exposed anorexia for what it was: a liar, a bully, and a beast.

Those days when I was fighting my eating disorder alone, scared and starving, I was sure that I would never see the light again. Those days when I was hiding from everyone what I was putting my body through, what I was doing to myself, I was sure that nobody on Earth had ever gone through what I was going through, I was sure no one would ever understand. Those days when I convinced myself I wasn't ill, even though my heartbeat was slow and shallow and I couldn't stand up without support, I thought that I would have to suffer like that for the rest of my life. I don't think I'll ever forget the hell I went through on my darkest days.

24 HOURS

Cold. That's the first thing I feel when I wake up. Not the refreshing chill of a bright summer morning, but the deep, perishing cold that chills you right to the bone. The kind of cold that makes you wonder if you'll ever be warm again. Despite that, there is that one blissful second, when I'm still drowsy with sleep, when I forget where I am. I could be anywhere – a five star hotel in a beautiful foreign country with people waiting on me hand and foot, a cosy country cottage somewhere on the coast where I can see the glistening sea from my window, a huge king-size bed in an enormous mansion with a library and a swimming pool. It doesn't really matter, as long as I'm anywhere but here. But as the cold sets in my hopes of a different life fade fast. I'm brought back to reality. A reality where I struggle through every waking moment, until I can close my eyes and escape from the torture of anorexia once again.

It takes me forever to pluck up the courage to free myself from my bed sheets. I cling on to what little protection they provide against the cold, and when I finally do give them up, I'm running to the heater to make sure it's on full blast for when I have to sacrifice my body to the frigid air and get dressed. Of course, it's the middle of August, and outside it's 23°C. To everyone around me it's a perfect summer's day – hot, but with a gentle breeze to temper the heat. But to me that breeze is like ice running through my skin. I head to the bathroom and inspect myself in the mirror, hoping to see something different than what's presented to me. A hope that will forever be within me, but will never be met. 'Just a little bit longer' I tell myself. 'Just keep pushing on a little bit longer'. Then I have the dreaded task of getting dressed. Taking off my pyjamas is the hardest part of my morning; I know when they've gone I'll be even colder than before, I'll be so close to tears that I have to bite my lip to keep them in. But soon I'll have the sweet relief of my uniform to keep me warm, although it hangs off my body like drapes.

I arrive at the hospital where I'm doing my placement, and I park in the car park a mile away from the entrance. My friend says he wants to walk instead of getting the bus, and reluctantly I agree. Something in my head is telling me that walking is better, healthier, but deep down I wonder if I will manage it, whether this will be the day that my weak and fragile legs simply give up on me. It takes a herculean amount of effort, but I make it to the hospital. There's just the two flights of stairs to navigate now – we could take the lift but the voice in my head is reprimanding me for even thinking of it. Every step is a challenge, every staircase a mountain to climb. When I make it to the top my legs are shaking and I don't think I could walk another step. But I have to. I'm not allowed to show weakness.

I know the next few hours are going to be spent on my tired, exhausted feet. I have some orange squash to fuel myself before I start, but it won't help. I'll still have to seek out walls to lean on, handles to hold to keep me upright. To make the impression that I'm okay. As for conversation, I will drift in and out, trying to follow what people are saying, but ultimately failing due to my ever-dwindling concentration. My brain is foggy, my thoughts are sparse, and when people ask me questions I try my best to produce an acceptable answer, but with next to no chance of succeeding. All I can think about is food. We go and see a patient and they have some grapes on their bed; what I would do to simply reach out and take one right now. It's agony. I listen to the clock ticking away, each second that passes gets me closer to the time when I'm allowed to eat again, when I'm allowed what my heart desires more than anything. I'm wobbling, I'm faint, and I'm weak, yet still I push on. This is my duty. This is my mission.

Lunchtime finally comes and I have to stop myself running to find a table. Watching everyone else unpack their lunchboxes has me salivating, but I will stay strong, I will not give in to the temptation of food. I take out my lunch and I know that this is the moment I have been waiting for. I have to eat so slowly to make sure I'm not finished before everyone else, but if I could, I would gobble down my lunch in a matter of seconds; I am so hungry. I take tiny bites, savouring each one as if it's the last thing I will ever eat. I know it will be hours before my body gets fuel again, and my brain knows it too. Part of me longs to go and get a chocolate bar to satiate the hunger, but another part of me rebukes the very thought.

Back on the ward for the afternoon, and I'm speaking with a patient. They're telling me their story, they're telling me the most private things in their life, but I can't hear them. The world is spinning and I feel faint. The voice in my head is saying 'don't you dare collapse on the ward, you pathetic excuse for a person', and I'm listening to it, because I know its words are the truth. I am pathetic. I feel awful yet I know exactly what to do to make it better – I have the cure right at my fingertips, but I'm just too scared to take it.

Back at home and I'm trying to do more studying, but I can't ignore the hunger pains or the desperate noises that are coming from my tummy. It's literally screaming out for food, but I will not honour it. I'm too strong-minded to give in that easily. My head congratulates me on making it this far. Hunger has turned into an achievement, fullness has become a failure. I want to get up from my desk and go for a lie down, but my weary, empty body fights against all movement. Just the effort of standing up is too much, so I sit in my chair, wondering how I will ever survive this. Wondering what more there is to come.

Eventually I crawl into bed, so relieved that the day is over. I know I'll have to do it all again tomorrow, but for now I can rest. I can finally allow my broken body to rest. Even though my bones are sticking into my mattress, and I can feel the beating of my heart, slower than the second hand on my clock, I feel okay. I've survived. I've made it through another 24 hours. But as my body starts to power down, my mind starts to come alive. In the darkness of my room I'm trapped with the thoughts racing around my head – why am I doing all of this? What am I really going to achieve? How will I ever escape this downward spiral of misery? And when my exhausted mind finally settles and allows me to drift off to sleep, I know it's only a matter of time until the fight begins once more.

EXPOSING
THE TRUTH

How are you meant to tell someone that you think you have an eating disorder? I came so close to telling my Mum so many times, but there was always something else going on. There was always something that anorexia could use as an excuse to delay the day that I started to defy it. First the cat died, then my Grandma was round for lunch, then my parents were going on holiday for the weekend. I never wanted to burden them with my problems, so I waited, and while I waited I lost more and more weight. The voice became stronger and I became weaker. The more time that passed the further I sank into the depths of my illness, and the harder it became to tell the truth.

But if it could, anorexia would come up with all

of the excuses in the world not to let someone else in on the secret. Anorexia would keep you as its prisoner forever, yet keep convincing you that you were free. I guess there's never really a convenient time to change someone's life by telling them you have an eating disorder, but any time is a good time to begin disobeying anorexia; any time is a good time for the war to commence.

I suppose something that makes my story slightly 'unusual,' is that I was the first person to realise that anorexia had taken hold of me. I was the one who reached out for support, I was the one who cried for help. My parents had no idea what was going on, in fact if I'd have told them that there was something wrong, I bet 'eating disorder' wouldn't have even crossed their minds. However being the first to know about the illness came with huge responsibility – it was up to me to expose the voice and share it's secrets with the world. It was up to me to fight through the screaming in my head, the threats that anorexia was throwing at me, and make sure that it was laid bare for all to see.

In some ways I wish someone else would have seen what was happening to me. I wish someone would have seen me getting weaker day by day until I was nothing. I wish someone would have seen me shrink into myself, disappearing first by millimetres, then by inches, then by miles. But anorexia does everything it can not to let that happen, it forces you to do the most secretive and devious things just to make sure that no one finds out about it. I suddenly found myself lying to everyone around me, just little white lies: 'I'm not hungry', 'I'm fine', 'I've already eaten', but with each lie came more shame and more guilt until it broke me.

When I thought about what I was doing, what I believed I was choosing to do, I was embarrassed. How could I let this happen? As a medical student, how could I be so irresponsible and careless? I was trusted to help look after patients yet I couldn't even look after myself. At first I didn't tell anyone because I was scared. I was scared that people would judge me; I was scared that people would be angry at me and not understand; I was scared that I would be deemed unworthy of help. After all, I believed that it was *my* decision not to eat, it was *my* decision to starve myself. I believed that I hadn't been suffering long enough to be properly ill. I believed that I was a fake, a fraud, that I hadn't lost enough weight to have 'proper' anorexia.

How I wish I would have told someone what was happening sooner. How I wish I would have realised that the more I was convinced I wasn't actually ill, the more hold anorexia had over me. The more I was convinced that I wasn't deserving of help, the more the eating disorder was controlling my mind and manipulating me. I know now that I was extremely unwell, but back then, when my brain was so starved and malnourished, it was difficult to comprehend the possibility that what I was doing was so terrifyingly dangerous. It was so hard to comprehend that while I was going on placement everyday, spending hours on my feet, then running miles at the weekend, I was actually dying. My body and my mind were failing. I seemed perfectly well on the outside, yet I was so gravely sick.

I didn't end up waiting for an ideal time to tell my Mum, I didn't wait for the perfect moment, I didn't even wait until I was ready, because I knew that I would never be ready. Anorexia would never be ready. I'd been through the lines in my head so many times that I'd come up with a million different ways of revealing the truth, but in the end none of them were right. In the end, my tears and my anguish told a much clearer story than my words ever could.

What really broke me that day, the two words that sent me so far into the most harrowing recesses of my mind, was something as simple as 'mashed potato'. When my Mum told me over the phone that she was going to cook mashed potato for me when I came home from university, little did she know that she was about to set off a cascade of terror, a fear burning so deep inside me that I gave up years of my life to it. I'd been avoiding potato for months, and the eating disorder became so overwhelmed that I couldn't think. It felt so threatened that it tore into me until I couldn't cope for a single second longer, and somehow, I finally began eating. I can't put into words what happened to me – it was like an out of body experience, like I was being controlled by an external force, but I was doing what I'd been scared to do for so long. I became more terrified with every bite, I became more detached from myself the longer it went on, but I was unstoppable. I was eating for my life.

At the time I thought I was crazy, I didn't know what was happening. But now I know that my brain was so malnourished that it went into survival mode – its sole aim was to find food, to save my life. There was nothing I could do to stop it; I didn't care what I was eating, I didn't care what it tasted like, all that mattered was that it was food. Finally, when I couldn't take a single bite more, I was brought back down to Earth. I knew in an instant that my worst nightmare had come true. I felt devastated, ashamed. The guilt was overwhelming. All I could think about was how to take back my actions, and I eventually concluded that my only option was to make myself sick, to rid my body of the thousands of calories that I'd just consumed. But right as I was about to go into the bathroom, my flatmate returned. At that point I knew. I knew that there was absolutely nothing I could do to make myself feel any better, and I was sick of it. I was sick of constantly feeling awful about myself, and I was so tired. I knew I couldn't go on anymore.

So I video-called my Mum. As soon as I saw her face on the screen I burst into tears; I didn't know what to say, I didn't know how to tell her that everything in my life was going so wrong. But eventually I managed it, the thing I'd been avoiding for so long. With anorexia screaming in my head and begging me to stop with every word, I fought through the noise and told her everything. I told her everything, but I refused to say the word 'anorexia'. In fact I wouldn't even say 'eating disorder': the terms felt so big, so scary, so official. But she knew. She knew straight away what we were dealing with, and she wasn't angry with me. She didn't think I was pathetic; she still loved me, and from that point on I knew we'd be fighting the battle together.

After I'd told my family the fight truly began. I knew I had to make an appointment with my GP, and although I only had to wait a week, it felt like a lifetime: when you're fighting all the time for survival, every second feels like an hour. I remember being sat in the waiting room full of apprehension, but also full of hope. Hope that I would be able to turn my life around. Hope that this would be the start of my healing, of my recovery. When I finally walked in to see the doctor, I knew I wasn't alone. Although my parents couldn't come with me to that first appointment, I knew that they were supporting me and pushing me on to get the help that I deserved.

But that appointment turned out to be inexplicably hard and upsetting. I was no longer just faced with the reality of having a serious and deadly illness, but I was also faced with the reality of having to take time off university to face it head on. For the first time I was angry. I was livid that anorexia could so easily take away this opportunity to fulfil my dreams. This opportunity that I'd worked so hard for. Surely I couldn't be that ill – I'd already managed to complete a physically and mentally demanding placement 5 days a week, I'd even achieved top marks in all of my coursework. I argued. I pushed to only have a couple of weeks off, because that's how long I thought it would take to recover. I tried to persuade anyone and everyone I thought had some power to stop me taking time off, but none of it worked – I was forced to move back home with my parents and confront my eating disorder head on.

Dear Jade,

This is going to be the biggest and toughest fight of your life. I know you don't feel like it right now, but asking for help was the bravest and strongest thing you ever did. Now you have to channel that strength and that bravery into recovery. Into claiming your life back.

There's a long and winding road ahead of you, too long to see the final destination. But have faith that the most beautiful destination is out there, waiting to welcome you into its arms. Many of your challenges are unknown, but don't let that give you fear – let it give you hope that you'll be able to overcome them, that they will merely be tiny bumps along your path.

I know that you're ready for this battle, I know that you are resilient enough and tough enough to withstand all of the blows that come your way. You may be scared, but know that you will never have to fight this alone. You may be frightened, but everyone is behind you, supporting you, carrying you when you're too weak and too tired to stand.

From this day on, you are a warrior. From this day on, you must fight with everything you have. From this day on, you must hold on to hope and never ever let go. Just stay strong, I know you can do this.

BREAKFAST

At first, the thought of recovery was exciting – I was going to be able to eat new foods, foods I'd been avoiding for so long. I believed that it would be quick and painless, I never thought for one second that it would be so hard, I never thought that it would require the sheer amount of bravery and resilience that I would soon have to find within myself. I was just waiting for reassurance, for anorexia's approval to eat. I believed that once the illness told me that it was okay to eat, that it was okay to nourish myself, it would be easy - I would be able to fill my body with energy, with the delicious food that I'd been missing out on. But I came to realise that it was never going to give me permission to eat; if I was waiting for its approval, I would have been waiting forever. So I had to grant myself permission to eat, I had to learn that being alive is permission enough to have food.

Being alive, simply living, meant that I deserved to nourish my body and feel no guilt or regret.

However the eating disorder told me that to prove myself, to prove my illness was real, I had to continue to lose weight. It told me that it was too soon to recover, too soon to let it go, and I believed it. I believed that I had to lose as much weight as possible, make myself as ill as possible to be worthy of treatment. It forced constant feelings of guilt onto me – guilt for using up NHS resources when I didn't deserve them; guilt for putting my family through absolute hell; guilt for seeking help when I didn't deserve help, when I wasn't ill enough. But somehow, through all of the noise and the hate, I managed to hang on to a tiny spark of hope, a tiny glimmer of light that pushed me to accept the help that I so desperately needed.

I began to see both a psychiatrist and a psychologist, an experience which I never imagined I would need. It was weird at first, opening up about what was going on in my head – I've never been very forthcoming about my feelings and emotions, and it felt unnatural and wrong to share them with a complete stranger. I struggled to describe how I felt, I struggled to understand what was running through my mind, but we worked together, and with their help and support I was able to slowly start increasing my food intake. For so long I'd deprived myself of so many foods, foods which I used to love, foods which I was experiencing such intense cravings for. The thought of those tastes, those textures, those smells filled me with a hope that burned strong inside me, which allowed me to take my first steps to recovery.

The very next day I ate breakfast – something which I'd been avoiding for so long - a forgotten venture, a huge challenge; but a challenge which I knew I had to face. As I placed my toast on the dining table, I did so with trembling hands. Fear gripped me so tightly that it seemed impossible for it to ever let me go, yet still I soldiered on. I wanted to turn around and run away with every fibre of my being, I wanted to run to safety, somewhere where I didn't have to suffer this anxiety. But with each and every bit of strength and bravery I could muster, with every last bit of fight within me, I faced my demons. I took my first bite, and it was wonderful. Terrifying, but wonderful. It was also so much harder than I ever could have ever imagined. It took every remaining bit of courage to carry on, to push through until the end, but somehow I managed it. Somehow I did what I'd been too scared to do for a long time, and I ate breakfast. I felt a very brief pang of pride before anorexia began to tear me down.

My heart started beating faster, I started to feel sick, and my whole body began to shake. The eating disorder told me that I was weak, it told me that I was greedy, it told me that I was a traitor. I'd disobeyed the voice; the voice which told me that my only option was to continue losing weight, the voice that was ruling my mind, telling me what was right and wrong. The anxiety that dominated my mind was unbearable and all I wanted to do was take everything back. Undo the damage that I'd done. Prove my loyalty to the eating disorder.

Anxiety plagued me the whole day, and it took all of my willpower to continue eating. The strong mind that had allowed me to restrict and resist food was now being put to the opposite use – it was forcing me to push through the pain and eat. Instead of seeing weight loss as an achievement, as I had been doing for so long, I now had to see weight gain as an achievement. Instead of not eating when I felt hungry, now I had to eat even when I felt full. Every couple of hours I would rush to the toilet and lift up my t-shirt to check that my stomach was still flat, to make sure that my ribs and my hip bones were still protruding from my fragile body. It was so illogical, believing that I might have gained weight just from one breakfast, but when I was trapped deep in my eating disorder, all logic was erased. I was terrified. I was terrified of what I'd done.

Day after day I pushed myself to eat my breakfast, and each day was harder than the last. It was such a small step towards recovery, but it brought with it enormous anxiety and distress. However somehow I managed to survive the onslaught of emotions careering around my mind, somehow I managed to slowly continue adding foods to my diet, despite the imminent threat of weight gain. But as I ate more, I struggled more. As my meals got bigger, so did my anxiety. On the surface it seemed like I was in a good place, it seemed like I was progressing well, but inside I was barely holding on. The more I ate the more I felt like a failure, like a traitor to the illness. It felt like I was losing, like I was finally giving up all of my willpower and succumbing to the temptation. Despite having some initial success in recovery, I was feeling more defeated by the day.

*'Even through the coldest winter and
the loneliest storm, she was fearless.'*

MENTAL
ILLNESS

Mental illnesses are secret worlds that trap you, force you to live a life that you hate, all the while seeing the worst in everything around you. You become detached from anything that makes you feel remotely happy, you exist on this Earth but you are living in a completely different reality. You see the light around you, but you only focus on the darkness. You're numb to real life, the only thing you feel is your mind bullying you, controlling your every move, your every decision. You have no emotions anymore, you've become a robot, following orders blindly from the relentless commander in your head.

It's confusing. It's overwhelming. It makes absolutely no sense yet somehow you know what it wants from you. It hurts you, but it leaves no mark. It rips you to shreds, yet somehow you still appear whole. It's all in your head, but nevertheless it's completely real. No one else can see your wounds, no one else can visualise your illness, and you'll convince yourself that you're imagining it. You'll convince yourself that you're a fraud, that your head is making everything up – all of your struggles and all of your hurt. But know that the voice is real. Know that you don't have to be showing physical illness to be suffering.

I think that people with mental illnesses become masters at disguising their pain. I think that they become brilliant actors and established liars, with the sole aim of deceiving everyone around them into believing that they're okay. Every time someone asks me how my day has been, I say 'fine', or even 'good', even if my day has involved me struggling to get out of bed, barely being able to take my medications, being exhausted to the point where I could hardly function. I always say my evening was 'okay', even when I spent it engaging in the most horrific eating disorder behaviours, even when I spent it a slave to anorexia.

But who am I really protecting? Am I trying to shield myself from the judgement of others when they find out about my mental illness, or am I trying to stop others feeling awkward when I'm brutally honest and tell them about what my life is really like behind closed doors?

There is such a taboo around words like 'depression', 'anorexia', 'self-harm', and countless others which make up significant parts of peoples' lives. There is such stigma and shame surrounding mental illness when it is just as valid and just as debilitating as physical illness. You don't hear people going around whispering about their asthma because they think they ought to be ashamed of it. You don't see people desperately trying to hide their plaster cast for a broken arm because they're worried people will judge them for their injury. So why should we hide? Why should we pretend that we aren't suffering when every minute of every day is a struggle?

FALLING

The first few weeks of my recovery were by far the hardest weeks I'd ever faced. I was supposed to be getting better, but I was rapidly falling back into the clutches of anorexia. For weeks I struggled in private. For weeks I pretended to be okay, while my mind was tearing me down.

I went to countless appointments at the eating disorders clinic, and I told people I wanted to recover because that's what I thought they wanted to hear. I told people I was aiming to put weight on because I knew that's what I was supposed to say. But these were other people's thoughts – unwelcome and imposing thoughts that I pretended to agree with, that I pretended to support. My thoughts weren't even close. My thoughts were completely focused on holding on to the eating disorder. Even though it was *my* idea to seek help, even though I brought my illness to the attention of everyone around me, I was stuck. I was stuck clinging on to a reality that was slowly killing me.

In the early days of my recovery, when I was full of hope and naivety, I made two goals – to eat cake on my birthday, and to eat Christmas dinner with my family. I was determined not to let anorexia take these days away from me, I swore I wouldn't let the voice win. But a couple of months later, a couple of months after embarking on my journey, both days had come and gone and I had achieved neither of my goals. I really thought I would be fixed by then. I prayed that I would be fixed by then, but I was even further away from freedom than when I started. I was travelling down the road to recovery in a pattern of one step forwards, two steps back. I would put on weight, then feel nothing but panic and end up losing it again - a horrendous cycle which could only lead to one outcome.

By Christmas I was defeated. I was losing my hair, my body was becoming covered in bruises, and I was too weak to properly cough. Imagine not having enough muscle in your chest to be able to clear your throat properly. At the most wonderful time of the year, I was failing, I was broken, I was so broken that I couldn't even scream out for help. I was trapped in my own head with nowhere to go, no route to escape. Any thoughts about recovery were gone, I was starting to accept that there was no way out, no way to come back from this.

I exercised in secret, restricted my food intake when no one was watching, and I was dishonest about it to everyone. I was deceiving all those who mattered to me yet the guilt wasn't enough to make me stop. I deteriorated even further and while the rational part of me tried to stop, tried to make a change, anorexia was praising me, it was telling me that I was doing so well and it was so very proud of me. No one mattered except the eating disorder, it was the most important thing in my life and it was with me wherever I went, whispering in my ear, telling me not to listen to anyone who was attempting to help me. I tried to ignore it, I tried to show it that I was the boss, but I had no energy left. The less I ate, the less strength I had to fight, and the voice just got louder and louder until it was deafening me. It was the only thing I could hear, the only thing I could feel. It seemed like it was the only thing inside me. I wasted away. My personality, my sense of humour, anything that I had left was taken by the eating disorder. I was nothing.

Despite my best efforts to hide my actions, they didn't go unnoticed. I knew that everyone suspected that things weren't going right but I refused to give up the voice. I rejected all claims that would expose the eating disorder and I remained loyal to the very thing that was ruining me. Until I couldn't keep it inside me any longer. Until in one of my sessions with my psychologist, on a cold and unforgiving December day, I decided that I'd had enough. I was done with being cold all the time, I was finished with sneaking around and hiding from everyone, I was ready to sacrifice control and relinquish any responsibility I had for my recovery to someone else. Anyone else who could help me out of this mess that I'd gotten myself into. Anyone who could save me from myself.

SINKING

I feel like I'm sinking. I've been thrown into a whirlpool, spiralling deeper and deeper, and now I have to attempt to drag myself back out with what little energy remains. It's just me and anorexia, trapped in war, fighting to the death. I'm desperately trying to cling to life, but anorexia rips it out of my hands. It deprives me of anything worth living for. All I can feel is the pain and misery enveloping me, causing me to sink further into this hell.

It's so dark. The light has been completely extinguished, giving no guide to the way home. My feet don't touch the ground, and I'm left floating in limbo, neither hitting the bottom nor breaking the surface. I thought the worst was close, but somehow I keep falling and falling, deeper than I ever thought I could go. All sound has been silenced, except for the screaming and shouting rattling my brain. I try to swim but I'm trapped. Trapped in cage which makes me feel small and insignificant, where no one can hear me cry.

Dear Jade,

I know that you feel angry and frustrated with yourself. I know that you feel like you're giving in to the voice too easily, but try to show yourself some compassion. You are doing the best you can to beat a powerful, unrelenting force; don't underestimate how much courage that takes.

It's okay if you can't always see the light at the end of the tunnel, because I know that you will keep on moving through the dark. It's okay if you feel too weak, too broken to carry on, because I have faith that you are strong, and you will battle through every challenge that comes your way. It's okay if you don't think you can beat this because I know that you will never stop fighting.

Even though recovery is so much harder than you ever thought it would be, you are not giving up, and that shows incredible resilience and determination. Your mind may be screaming otherwise, but you don't deserve to suffer, and you don't deserve to be in pain.

You have taken the first steps to recovery, now you just have to keep moving forward. Whether you run, or whether you crawl, just keep looking ahead and going in the right direction.

THE ILLNESS
AND ME

One thing that I really struggled with throughout my recovery was the differentiation between myself and the eating disorder. At the start everything felt all mixed together, like combining skittles and M&Ms in one bowl – everything looks the same, but really you have two complete opposites. The same was true of the thoughts and feelings in my head: I was the anorexia and the anorexia was me. We were one and the same, the lines between us blurred until we could no longer be distinguished as ourselves.

But eventually I learnt to see the divide between us. We may look the same, we may sound the same, but I am NOT anorexia. Anorexia is a monstrous beast who sets out to ruin lives, whereas I am just a young woman trying my best to live a good and happy life. For so long I had been convinced that I was an awful person, that the thoughts that came from my own head were pathetic and true. I trusted my mind to show me the right way to live and I followed its guidance without question, to the point where I was blind to the possibility that anything could be amiss. But when the idea that anorexia could be separate from myself was planted in my brain, it was a wild possibility that I began to lay my hopes on. I knew that if it was true, this could be my escape.

Once I started to see the illness as something separate from myself, I was able to begin defying it in little ways: I could acknowledge that the shouting in my head telling me to go for a longer walk wasn't me. It wasn't normal, it wasn't rational, and most importantly, it wasn't right. So I'd become rebellious and take the short route. When my mind was telling me to choose an apple at snack instead of some biscuits I took time out to think about which I'd prefer in my heart, and when the answer was biscuits, I would suffer the anxiety because it meant that anorexia had taken a hit. I know that these small victories seem insignificant, but to me they meant the world. To me they meant that I was beating the voice. At the start of my recovery I began to take every thought as a challenge, and every decision as an opportunity to make myself stronger, and the voice weaker.

But over time anorexia took on a personality all of its own. I allowed it to become someone who had its own voice, someone who I was allowing to bully me, to ruin me. Anorexia was my best friend and my nemesis, my companion and my biggest enemy. I could picture it in my head, controlling my thoughts and my future, hiding so that it couldn't be seen and I began to doubt whether it existed at all. I was sure that nobody would ever believe me if I told them about this separate entity inside me, but I wasn't the only one suffering with this invasion, it happens to all kinds of people: men, women, old people, young people, Mums, Dads, sisters, brothers, nurses, university lecturers, beauticians, shop assistants, office workers, and everyone in between. Eating disorders don't discriminate, and although mental illness is lonely, we are never alone. We are an army fighting for our lives. Fighting to eradicate this monster.

It's rather unsettling at first, not being able to trust your own mind. Your mind, your thoughts, your opinions, are what make you who you are. So when something evil hijacks your brain with its hate and fear, it's hard to accept that those thoughts aren't you. It's hard to accept that you will act on those thoughts and be ashamed of yourself later for feeling like you gave in so easily. You will believe these thoughts without question, and argue against logical reasoning to the point where you start to convince yourself that the voice is right. You will be extremely uncomfortable with the things running through your head and pretend that everything is okay, when really you're breaking with the effort it takes to appear 'normal'.

The only thing I found harder than having these thoughts from the voice, was trying to explain them to other people. Sometimes I couldn't put into words what was going on in my mind, and sometimes I was simply too embarrassed to say them out loud. I didn't believe anyone else had ever felt how I felt. I thought I was an anomaly, the only one who was being tortured by her own mind. Telling someone I couldn't eat a carrot because I believed that it was going to make me put on weight made me feel stupid. Telling someone I had to park my car further away from the entrance so I could burn extra calories walking made me feel completely humiliated. But I know that the real me, the real Jade, she doesn't care how many steps I do each day, and I know that realistically, she knows that eating a carrot will not cause her to gain weight.

It's exhausting, having to stop and analyse each and every thought, each feeling that runs through your head. It's exhausting having to constantly fight against your own mind, against this unseen force that exists only inside your head. It's exhausting, but it's courageous. It's tiring, but it is so, so brave.

It's not just thoughts on food and exercise anorexia injected into my brain - it took over my whole life. Every little thing I did, everything I felt was contaminated by the illness. Here are some more things it told me:

- I'm such a burden that everyone's fed up with me
- No one could possibly love me because I'm an awful person
- I'm not good enough for this world and I shouldn't be here
- I shouldn't have treatment for my eating disorder because it's taking resources that I don't deserve away from those who are more ill than me
- I'm a pathetic excuse for a human and I can't do anything right
- Everyone around me is beautiful and kind and I'm completely self-absorbed
- I don't deserve to buy myself nice things, like new clothes, because I haven't done anything to earn them
- I'll never succeed in life and I'll always be a failure

- Whatever I do, I'll end up letting everyone in my life down
- Everybody secretly hates me, and they're talking about me behind my back

Thinking of all these things that I once believed to be true, I have one thing, and one thing only to say to anorexia: I feel sorry for you. You get strength from tearing other people down and it's pathetic. You feel happy when you make other people suffer and it's pitiful. You will never ever win because I no longer believe anything you tell me. I no longer need you. I am determined to get rid of you for good, and I won't let you ruin my life any longer. I am so much more than you'll ever be, and I deserve so much more than your lies and your hate. You can't touch me anymore, I am determined to live a life without an eating disorder, without you constantly hanging on to me. I am determined to be free.

To Anorexia,

I want my life back. This isn't me asking for my life back, this is me telling you I'm taking my life back. You have taken so much from me: it's your fault I've had to take time off University, it's your fault my parents are having to take me to countless appointments. It's you that's responsible for ruining things, not me. Although you did manage to convince me for some time that it was my fault, I can see through you now.

You've made me hit rock bottom. You've made me cry in bed and never want to get up. You've made me so tired and weak that I don't take care of myself. You've put the idea in my head that nothing matters anymore. You've made my hair fall out in clumps and given me loose and dry skin. You've made it so that my broken body will no longer fit into any clothes. You've given me bruises all down my legs and hips, even huge ones on my bum from where I've simply sat on the toilet. You've made me so cold that I've wanted to cry because it's impossible to get warm. You've made me so bony that it's uncomfortable to sit on a chair or even to lie in bed. You've made me miss out on countless opportunities with friends and family. You've made me feel so guilty about eating an extra piece of broccoli that I did laps around the living room.

The worst part is that you've managed to convince

me for so long that I wasn't ill – that this was all normal.

Well you're not in control anymore. I'm going to eat the chocolate, and cake, and cheese, and pasta. Maybe not today, or tomorrow, but eventually it will happen and when it does I will laugh. I will laugh at you because you're pathetic.

I don't know why you chose to haunt me, but it didn't work, did it? You didn't last long before I figured out what you were up to, and I won't just get rid of you. I will destroy you. You chose the wrong person to mess with and I will prove that.

P.S. Fuck off

HOSPITAL

Months after I started to recover, I was still completely and utterly trapped in my illness. Despite my initial success in early recovery, I had continued to deteriorate and the voice was stronger than ever. I gave up trying to regain control of my own mind, I gave up doing things on my own terms, and I was admitted to a general hospital. At my most weak and vulnerable, I was losing the unwavering support of having my family around me, and the comfort and safety of my home. I was losing any tiny bits of progress that I'd managed to make and I was being fed through a tube. It was degrading, it was undignified, and it was undoubtedly the worst experience of my life.

Surely anorexia had what it wanted now. Surely forcing me into this position was enough to make it stop torturing me, but it stayed strong. I knew that I just had to stay even stronger.

The first night that I slept in a hospital bed I cried and cried until I had no tears left. What had my life come to? I didn't recognise the person in my body anymore, in fact I didn't even recognise my body. I would look in the mirror and see a ghost staring back at me. A pale, worn-out, inhuman ghost. I was completely detached from reality. The person living my life wasn't Jade, it was anorexia. Anorexia took up so much of my mind that there wasn't room for anything else. There wasn't room for hope, and there wasn't room for happiness. Every night while I was being pumped full of calories through my tube the eating disorder would scream and shout at me for letting the staff feed me, for letting the staff save my life. It was livid. It was furious. I lived day to day just pushing through the hours trying to think of anything but food, anything but the eating disorder. More often than not I ended up spending my time fantasising about an alternative life. A life where anorexia didn't exist and I was back at university, living my life independently and free. Living the life I deserved to have.

On a particularly hard night during my hospital stay, I lay in bed and spent hours pulling out my hair. My beautiful hair which I refused to get cut, which broke my heart every time big clumps fell out into my hands when I brushed it. But I didn't care - in that moment I just wanted to hurt. The elderly lady in the bed opposite me attempted to provide comfort, but comfort wasn't what I needed. I needed peace, I needed rest, I just needed everything to go away.

The tears that I shed that night left a small stain on my pillow. You could hardly see it but somehow I knew, when I woke up in the morning after a long and tortuous night, where to look. And I saw not a mark a mark of bravery for carrying on, nor a mark of strength for refusing to give up, but a mark of sorrow. I saw my troubles and my distress, a stark reminder of the hell that I was facing every minute of every day.

Every afternoon that I spent on that ward, I would count down the minutes until visiting time, when my family would come and distract me from the pain, from the agony of being in hospital. I counted down the minutes until I could be wrapped up in my Mum's arms, protected and safe from harm, if only for a few minutes. Every single night I felt blessed to be tucked into bed by my parents, to receive a kiss on the head – a promise to love me always, and forever stand by my side.

But however much these visits kept me going, however much I loved and appreciated my family; I always felt so much pressure to make the time that we spent together perfect, to make each and every visit worthwhile. I felt like I had to keep the conversation going when I was too tired and too fatigued to talk. I had to pretend that I was coping when all that I'd done that day was cry. I had to pretend that everything was fine when I was falling apart, so that they wouldn't go home in tears themselves.

I never admitted it to them, and I even refused to admit it to myself, but I came to resent those afternoons. Those afternoons where I felt pressure to be the perfect hostess, where I felt like everyone was expecting more from me than I was able to give. On a particularly hard day, I shouted at my Dad to stop visiting me. I shouted at him to leave me alone when I needed his love more than anything, when all I needed in that moment was for him to comfort me and tell me that everything was going to be okay.

I felt horrendously guilty, I felt like I was a despicable and nasty person, but it was all anorexia. It was the illness, poisoning my brain, twisting my mind, squeezing every feeling of happiness out of my body. It was exhaustion, it was the effects of being so weak and weary, and it was the eating disorder constantly beating me down until I had nothing left to give. It was torture, but I knew it was torture for my family too.

It's only looking back now that I see the extent of the damage that anorexia was doing to me. It's only now that I can appreciate just how ill I was, and just how close I came to giving in to the voice. Each afternoon when my Mum walked onto the ward I begged her to take me up to the top of the hospital so I could look out of the windows at the world below. It reminded me that life was still happening, the world kept turning, although for me it felt like everything had been halted.

The nurses insisted that if I was going off the ward I had to be in a wheelchair. I was considered too poorly to walk, I was considered at risk of falls because of how weak I was. And yet I still didn't feel ill enough. Every four hours when I had my blood pressure taken I got a stark reminder of my dire physical situation, but anorexia didn't care – the illness loved it. It treated it like a competition with itself: how low would my blood pressure be today? Can I set a record for my lowest ever reading? The more the nurses became concerned, the more the illness told me how proud it was of me. The lower my blood pressure the bigger the thrill that went through my body. I was becoming more and more ill by the day, but the anorexia was thriving.

I often find myself wondering what it was like for others to see me in that condition – did they see the pain I was going through? Did they see my personality fall away until I was nothing? Were they worried about me? Were they scared about what I was doing to my body? Only when I look back can I appreciate how hard it must be to see someone you love slipping away little by little until you feel like you've lost them forever.

One evening at the end of visiting hours, I sent my Mum home with a task: try and find some pyjama shorts that would fit me. I didn't care how ugly they were, I didn't care whether they were for boys or girls or men or women, I just needed something to wear that wouldn't fall down, that would stay up on my frail, bony body. A couple of days later she had completed her mission; she walked in holding a shopping bag and handed me my shorts so I could go and try them on. I pulled them out of the bag and knew instantly that they were from the children's section, but to be honest I didn't really expect anything else. But as I pulled them on and found that they fit me perfectly, I caught a glimpse of the size.

These shorts that my Mum had looked at and thought would fit me, these shorts which hugged my waist perfectly; they were meant for a young child. They were meant to be worn by a five year old. I don't normally take much notice of clothing sizes – I know that they vary widely, and I know that they're unreliable and cannot possibly be compared between shops, but something told me that a 20 year old fitting into these shorts wasn't normal. My first thought was that I should be ashamed, I thought that I ought to be embarrassed, but that didn't last long before the eating disorder kicked in with its pride and glory. It just loved the fact that not only did these shorts fit me, but my Mum bought them with the belief that I'd fit into them, meaning that she thought I was skinny. Someone else saw me, someone else saw my body and thought that I was thin. It was a victory for anorexia, but a wake-up call for me - I was trapped in this child's body. I no longer felt like a grown up, I no longer felt like a woman.

'She knew a storm was coming. But instead of retreating, she closed her eyes and stepped into the rain, knowing that it would only help her to grow.'

TUBES

I n hospital I was kept safe, I was kept alive with tubes pumping me full of calories and needles breaking my delicate skin every day. But anorexia was kept alive too. The ignorance surrounding eating disorders gave anorexia food to thrive and although I was saved physically, mentally I was drowning.

'Are you not hungry enough to eat yet?' 'Are you being fed through a tube because you don't like the hospital food?' 'The whole point of recovery is to eat, you know.' Just some of the damaging comments tossed at me by the people who were supposed to be making me feel better.

'She doesn't deserve to be here and get treatment. She chose to be ill.' An overheard conversation from the other patients in my bay when they thought I was fast asleep. How I wish I'd been asleep and dreaming of paradise, instead of hearing confirmation that everything I believed was true. Instead of giving anorexia more reason to tell me that I'd brought all of this on myself. I no longer just had the guilt of taking in calories to contend with: the illness made me feel even more guilty for being in hospital, I felt guilty for being alive. I didn't deserve to take up one of the precious beds because I thought that others needed it more than me. I felt like a burden on the NHS, our wonderful NHS which was giving me so much help and support, yet I didn't deserve it one bit. The eating disorder was in my head all of the time, berating me for being so selfish, so inconsiderate. The one time when I knew I needed to be kind to myself, to forgive myself, I was attacking myself for something which wasn't my fault. I was attacking myself for falling ill.

Being fed through a tube I didn't have to worry about what I was eating anymore. I didn't have to worry about whether I was putting too much spread on my toast, or too much milk in my cereal. I could let someone else do the worrying for once, it was terrifying but I relinquished control and I put my trust into the experts. Until I couldn't trust them anymore.

I meticulously kept track of how many calories were being pushed into me each night – my eating disorder still couldn't let go of the obsessive calorie counting. I knew off by heart the times that the pump should be switched on and when it would beep in the early hours of the morning to tell me that it had finished its job. So one morning a couple of weeks into my hospital stay, when I woke up at 08:00am and the machine was still pumping, I went stiff. My body was paralysed with fear and I knew in that moment that the pump hadn't been set right. I knew that I'd been given far more through my tube than I was supposed to have, and it honestly felt like my world would end. I was clueless as to how I could carry on when disaster had struck. The feelings that consumed me were bigger, scarier than ever. I thought I was going to die from the panic and the pain.

Eventually I managed to hammer my buzzer for the nurses to come and sort it out, but I knew in my heart that the worst had already happened. Physically I was fine, but psychologically I was traumatised. I cried and cried in bed, and no one could comfort me because to them my crying was a mystery. They had no idea why I was so upset over a few calories. So I was left alone with my mind, catastrophising the amount of weight I would gain from this mistake. When my psychiatrist came to see me I begged him to let me go home, but to no avail. I was stuck here, stuck on this miserable hospital ward with no life or joy left inside me. I had no choice left but to continue trusting these people with my life.

A few days later I remember vividly waking up and thinking about the rest of the people on my university course starting their new placements. This was the day that I had begged to go back to university when I was first diagnosed. This was the day that I was sure I would be free of my eating disorder, free of the weights dragging me down. Yet instead of being with my friends and colleagues at medical school, I was in hospital, more poorly than ever. It should have been a wake-up call, but anorexia wouldn't allow that: it was too thrilled, too delighted that I was still stuck in its chains. It was still vowing to torture me until I broke.

Thankfully, when a bed in a specialist eating disorder inpatient unit became available I was moved there. I was much further away from my family and everything I knew, but I was finally going to get the help and support that I'd desperately needed for so long. I was scared, I was scared of being the biggest person there, I was scared of being the healthiest person there, and I was scared I'd eat the most.

I was so nervous at the prospect of meeting other people with eating disorders. As anorexia is an insanely competitive illness, it's constantly striving to be the 'best'. The best at losing weight, the best at being skinny, the best at starving you. On the run-up to going to the specialist unit, I knew I wasn't going to be the 'best' anymore, and that scared me more than anything. I felt like I was going to be the odd one out, the impostor, and I feared that my illness would be exposed as being 'fake'. I was worried about hating the other patients, and them hating me because of our illnesses competing, but I knew I had to go. I knew I had to put a brave face on, and step into the unknown.

Dear Jade,

Anorexia has so many weapons it will use against you in this battle – doubt, insecurity, fear. But believe it or not, you have a weapon stronger than all of those things put together. You possess something so special and so pure that it will win every single time if you find it within yourself.

Love.

Anorexia can't feel love. In fact it forbids it. It even hides it from you, tries to steal it away, destroy it. But love, whatever form it comes in, is indestructible. Anorexia will never succeed because love is strong, and love is resilient, and NOTHING can ever take that away from you.

Love gives you a determination to survive. Love gives you the power to forgive the world for putting you through all of this suffering. Love gives you an anaesthetic to numb the pain that is tearing you apart, and an antidote to the poison in your mind.

It can hurt, it can amplify the guilt screaming at you, but sometimes we have to suffer that pain to heal.

You have so many people who love you. You are allowed to love yourself, your body, your mind, and you are allowed to show your love for other people. Let it pour out of you until it drowns out everything else. Let it heal you until you become whole again.

Love prevails, even when you think you don't deserve

to be loved.

Love travels across boundaries, across borders, and is still felt as strongly as if it were standing right next to you.

Love wraps you in warmth, and whispers that everything will be alright, even when you can't believe it yourself.

You are loved. Now you just need to find it in you to love yourself. Embrace everything that makes you you, and don't leave a doubt in your mind that you are worthy of all of the love in the world. Love will set you free. It is freedom and hope rolled into one. It is a reminder of what you have to fight for, and what you stand to lose if you give up too easily.

THE INPATIENT UNIT

Arriving at the inpatient unit and stepping through the front door after already spending so long in hospital, my heart felt like it was beating out of my chest. But I needn't have worried - I was instantly greeted with warmth and welcome. Instead of being referred to as '6-4' (my bed number on the general ward), I was called Jade. I was respected, I was more than just an illness they had to treat, I was a person.

I was shown to my room, and I instantly noticed that there were no mirrors, not even in the bathrooms – nothing to amplify the distress I was already in. There were no proper coat hooks, window handles, door handles, wardrobe railings, as they were considered to be ligature risks. Any sharp items in my possession were taken off me and kept safe so I wouldn't fall victim to any urges to self-harm. I was given a pressure cushion to sit on so that my bum didn't hurt anymore. I was spoken to with kindness and caring. More than just that, I was spoken to with understanding. I felt cared for, I felt safe. I'm not saying that I enjoyed being in hospital – far from it. I just think that after my stint on a general ward the specialist unit was a welcome improvement. The specialist unit was so much better equipped to help me, to heal me.

My eating disorder was prepared to loathe the other patients. It was ready to fight against them every step of the way to prove itself, but that plan went out of the window straight away. As soon as I met everyone else I realised that they were just as broken as me. They were just as lost and confused as I was, trying to scramble their way through their own illness to get to see the light on the other side. I realised that we were all in this together, and I think that when you're going through hell, you would do anything at all to help somebody else who's going through hell with you. It didn't matter that all of our stories were different, and it didn't matter who I was or where I came from, I was not made to feel fake, and I was not made to feel invalid; I was made to feel loved and appreciated.

Being in the unit made it feel like the world had stood still - nothing else mattered but my health and wellbeing. I was finally in the right place, I was finally in the place that I was sure was going to cure me. At the start I had no formal therapy, and I was too ill to join in with many of the activities; but that was okay. Just allowing my body and mind to rest, just lying on the sofa in front of the television was healing in itself. I allowed myself to sleep during the day. I allowed myself to do things that I enjoyed – reading, painting, writing. I learnt that rest is so vital to recovery. I learnt that to rest is okay. I learnt the importance of self-care and just taking a break.

But it wasn't long before I was forced to confront my worst fear head on, in the form of a jacket potato with cheese and beans. I knew that this was where the excruciatingly hard work would begin. This was why I was here, not just to watch television and relax. My mind began to race, and my thoughts became completely dominated by the eating disorder. If I had to describe what I was feeling in that moment, I don't think I'd be able to – so many emotions were consuming me, a tornado of fear and dread. After being tube-fed for the last month I was being thrown into the deep end, and I just prayed that I wouldn't sink.

As I walked on shaking legs into the dining room, I took in the sights and the smells, and suddenly

I was hungrier than I'd ever been. Suddenly I was ravenous and it was all I could do to stop myself devouring what was in front of me. Although I was exceptionally nervous, I started to recognise sparks of excitement fighting through the fog in my head. I started to realise that this was what I'd been waiting for. I believed that anorexia was finally giving me permission to eat. I believed that I was finally ill enough, finally skinny enough for the eating disorder, and this was the permission that I'd been unknowingly holding on for, which I'd been so desperate to find for so long. I looked around and the other patients were eating. The other patients were soldiers, battling through the war ripping through their minds, and I decided in that moment to do the same. I decided to fight.

I ate so slowly; I was the last at the table even though my portion was smaller than everyone else's. After not eating for so long I was trying to savour the wonderful yet forgotten flavours, I was trying to discern every different texture that I possibly could. I wouldn't cut up the food on my plate or get more food on my fork while I was chewing because I needed to focus all of my attention on the taste of what I already had. I cut up my food into the tiniest pieces so that it would last longer, sometimes eating baked beans one at a time. Every mouthful was wondrous yet contaminated with guilt. Eventually my plate was clean, I'd passed my first test with flying colours; and although the eating disorder thoughts were strong, I knew that I'd just proven myself to be even stronger.

I'd made a good start, in fact I'd made a brilliant start, but it wasn't long before anorexia caught up with me. The adrenaline rush and thrill of the first day, of getting a taste of food again was fading, and pretty soon she convinced me that what I did wasn't just wrong, it was abhorrent. As I completed more meals over the next few days her reign became ever more powerful. She had allowed me a second of respite but now I was paying for it. Now I was suffering. The worst came less than a week after I had arrived at the inpatient unit. The worst came after I ate half a portion of rhubarb crumble for dessert after my tea. An astounding victory for me, but the beginning of a long and damaging rampage for anorexia.

It began with two words: two little words that changed my whole mindset. Two little words from the nurse that had sat with me and seen me struggle for hours over my tea, that sent me spiralling downwards faster than I ever thought possible. 'Well done'. Simple words with a well-intended meaning. Simple words that I should have accepted feeling proud of myself, but instead made me crumble to the ground and surrender to my eating disorder. As soon as the words were in the air a darkness clouded my mind – it was like anorexia was getting ready to attack, to knock me down and leave me pleading for mercy. All because somebody had said 'well done', all because someone thought that I was doing well.

The thing is, anything good, anything positive that I managed to achieve meant that I was putting anorexia's existence in danger. If I was doing well, it meant that anorexia was failing, and if there's one thing anorexia hates, it's to fail. So it told me that I was doing too well. It told me that doing well was a bad thing – everyone would hate me if I did well and no one would believe that I was ill. Again, that feeling of being a fake, of my illness not being real dominated my thinking. It told me that if I continued like I had been I'd recover too quickly, I'd gain weight too quickly. The eating disorder was determined to drag this out until the very end. It was determined that if it was to be brought down, it would bring me down too. It was determined to break me before I could beat it.

It was evil. The eating disorder abused me and taunted me that night until I ran to my bedroom sobbing, until I would have done anything to escape the torment that was raging through my mind. I couldn't think straight, I was devastated by what I'd done. I thought that I would never survive that feeling, that level of mental torture. I wanted the darkness to swallow me up, to gift me salvation from the pain. I hoped with everything I had that this was a dream, that I would wake up from the nightmare soon, but instead of being saved, I was subjected to even more distress in the form of my supper.

I'd been crying for hours and I was exhausted, I had nothing left to give when I was called to the dining room for my evening glass of milk. I sat in my seat and sobbed hysterically while the staff tried to make me drink. I screamed, I screamed at them that I wouldn't have the milk, yet they persisted. Tears were streaming down my face and I couldn't have stopped them if I'd tried. It felt impossible, just getting through the next minute felt impossible. But somehow, through all of the tears and all of the torment, I just about managed to pull through. I survived when I thought that survival wasn't an option, and for that I am proud.

I may not have drunk the milk, but I was proud of myself for turning up and trying. I may have gone to bed never wanting to wake up, but I'm proud of myself for getting up and carrying on the following morning. Most of all I am proud of myself for continuing my life, when in that moment all I wanted to do was die.

But that one comment had affected me so badly that I no longer wanted to recover. I knew that I was going to feel that horrific every time I rebelled against the illness. I knew that I never wanted to hear any form of praise again unless it was from the eating disorder, so I avoided it at all costs. I avoided it by starting to leave increasing amounts of food on my plate: I started to refuse snacks, and I started to rebel against the people who were trying to give me back my life. I still felt awful about what I was eating, but the bursts of joy from anorexia provided me temporary relief from the pain. Do I wish now I could go back in time and keep up the good work that I'd started? Of course I do. Do I wish I would have just swallowed my fears and sat at the table for hours working through a sandwich? Yes – I wish more than anything that I would have held on just a little longer, just found a little more strength inside me.

As I got worse and worse I was told I needed to put more effort in and I was threatened with supplements – drinks with hundreds of calories in them that would replace my meals - but anorexia saw this as a triumph. The more I was struggling, the more it told me that I was strong and the more it applauded me. I was forced to sit in front of hundreds of calories while sobbing into my meals. When they made me sit at the table in front of a yoghurt with jam in it, I started to hyperventilate. The panic that was consuming me at the mere thought of eating a yoghurt was indescribable. I was a mess, but anorexia thrived off the pain that I was going through. It fed on my fear and insecurities, and when I thought it couldn't get any stronger, it just kept growing and growing. Although I wanted to recover, my mind still wasn't done being ill. Even after all this time, the eating disorder still wasn't ready to leave. This was my last hope, the final chance for anyone to save me, and I was falling further and further into despair.

FAMILY

Anorexia doesn't like to be shared. It wants to be the only thing in your life, it wants to push away anything and anyone who might jeopardise your commitment to it.

Anorexia didn't want me to love my parents, it didn't want me to have friends, it wanted me to hate everyone around me, especially those who were trying to help. An eating disorder can put strain on even the strongest of relationships, yet for me those relationships were an essential and vital part of my recovery. When I couldn't muster up enough motivation to recover for myself, my family became my reason. I knew I was putting them through hell, having to watch me fade away in front of them, but I also knew that I could save them, and I knew that I was the only one who had that power. It was up to me to rescue those who loved me from becoming victims of the eating disorder too.

The hardest times were when I didn't feel loved, when I didn't feel worthy of love. Who was I recovering for then? I was sure that no one cared about me, no one was bothered about me or my illness, I felt totally alone in this world. But I know now that there was never a time when I wasn't loved. There were plenty of times when anorexia tried to make me believe otherwise, but it was all lies.

When I first told my parents about my eating disorder, I expected a lack of understanding, and I was fine with that; how could I expect them to understand it if I couldn't even understand it myself? But I was surprised to be proven wrong. My worst nightmare was returning home to be forced to eat everything that scared me the most. I thought I'd find the fridge stocked with my favourite chocolate bars, the cupboards overflowing with treats to 'fatten me up', but instead of ignorance, I got nothing less than unconditional love and acceptance. I got an army to stand up and fight alongside me. Me, my Mum, my Dad, my sister, and my brother all battling together to drive this unwelcome force from our home and from our lives.

At first we were strong, at first we were invincible, but as we all became worn down and tired, anorexia became more prominent inside me and I no longer wanted an army; I wanted to surrender to the illness. Every time someone encouraged me to eat my mind would tell me that they were trying to sabotage my life. Every time someone tried to be kind I would push them away, thinking that they were just pretending or they were acting out of pity.

More than once I acted horrifically towards people who were just trying to show me affection, who were caring for me from the bottom of their heart. I would shout and I would scream. I would tell them to stop talking to me, to leave me alone. I would lash out and tear into them when they were just trying to help, to show me love.

I could continue to completely blame myself for my actions and live with horrendous guilt, or I could acknowledge anorexia's role in all of this heartache. I'm not using the eating disorder to absolve me from taking responsibility for my actions, but it helps to provide an explanation as to why I hurt the very people who loved me the most. I was no longer myself, I no longer had a personality. My starved brain was barely functioning, it was barely alive. The idea that these people had intentions other than to see me healthy and happy came completely from the fear of the eating disorder. The fear that the eating disorder had of the abandonment that stemmed from my recovery.

When my Dad came to visit me in the hospital and I shouted at him to leave me alone and stop coming, it may have been my body carrying out the actions, but the intent was all from anorexia. Although he didn't understand at the time, and it upset him greatly, I hope that he now knows that it was the monster taking over my mind that shot anger and aggression towards him, not me. If I could apologise for the monster's actions I would give him a thousand sorrys, and it still wouldn't be enough to show him how much I despise what I said.

When I refused to eat and got angry with my Mum for trying to encourage me, I wish she knew my anger was misplaced. I wish she knew that it was anorexia getting angry at the thought of me getting better, I knew deep down that her actions came from love and concern for my health.

When I was miserable and bought no joy to our home, I wish my sister knew that the little gestures she gifted me meant the world. Taking me to the cinema, buying me the fluffiest blanket ever to keep me warm, and being someone who would always be there should I ever need some sisterly advice.

I wish my brother will forgive me in the future for being a huge burden on everyone, and having such a massive impact on the family when he should have been getting support in his first year of university.

I will forever be more grateful than I could ever express to everyone who stuck by me through my darkest times. I will forever be indebted to those who loved me, when my actions meant that I did not deserve to be loved. I will forever appreciate and adore those people who always found the right thing to say, when I thought that nothing anyone could say would make me feel better. I'm so lucky that I had such a strong support network throughout my illness when I know that many people don't. I may be irritable with them at times, and anorexia may not always fully appreciate them, but I want them to know how blessed and fortunate I feel to have people forever by my side. Forever fighting my corner.

To our daughter Jade,

When you were a toddler you would always make us smile, a right little comedian. You were always on the go, always happy, and very inquisitive.

When you told us the news that you were struggling with an eating disorder our lives changed. We knew in an instant that this, as a family, was going to be the hardest thing we had ever faced.

When you were tube-fed in hospital, when we dropped you off at the eating disorder unit, and when you had to be readmitted, you faced everything that was thrown at you with the utmost bravery.

You astonish us with your strength and resilience, and your determination to beat your eating disorder and return to your studies.

You're one of the bravest people we know. Keep fighting this and know that we have your back, always. We love you more than words can say.

Love From Mum and Dad xx

SUPPLEMENTS

When I think back to my first weeks on the inpatient unit I remember being stood still, stuck in the mud with no energy to move. There was no light in the dark, no sunshine in the storm. Every time I tried to move forward I fell off the edge and ended up lower and more battered than I'd been before. Despite being surrounded by people who knew what I was going through, whose job it was to help me and support me, anorexia was still convincing me that it was the only one I would ever need.

I knew that the only way I could get out of the unit and go home was to eat, yet it still wasn't happening. Every single meal I was still fighting against the illness in a haze of anger. It was angry at me for eating too much, and I was angry at myself for not eating enough. I was watching other patients struggling and felt like I had to struggle too. I was listening to screams of terror from people being restrained and wondering if I was giving in too easily. I was affected by everything happening around me and I was questioning everything I did, every decision that I made.

I would battle through the horrendous thoughts and the unwavering guilt for hours. One of my earliest meals on the unit – a quarter of a plate of pasta, took me almost two hours to complete. I can't describe the embarrassment within me when the dining room consisted of just me and a staff member watching me eat, the shame when people would start cleaning the tables around me, signalling the end of the meal yet I was barely half way through. But it was just one more way that the illness had me trapped, just one more way that it kept me in its clutches.

The longer I sat in front of the food, the louder and more vicious the voices became. They chanted insults at me, they bullied me until I could bear it no longer and I surrendered. I was drained, I was shaky, I was tired of fighting. I thought that things would get easier the more times I tried, I thought I would learn to ignore the voice a little better, but I was so wrong. Day after day things got harder. Day after day anorexia was gaining strength, while mine was fading away. Each meal was worse than the one before, each bite took more courage than the last.

Eventually it all bubbled up inside me and became too much. I hit a wall and knew that there was no way forward. I was too busy trying to be the 'perfect anorexic' but there was no such thing. The illness was constantly telling me that 'someone with real anorexia wouldn't eat that', or 'someone really suffering wouldn't be laughing at the dinner table'. I spent all of my time trying to prove to myself that my illness was real, and meanwhile I was pushing my mind deeper and deeper into the eating disorder.

I spent almost all of my time at the dinner table, breaking with the sheer determination that it took to persevere through the greatest struggle of my life. I'd just left the table after one fight and almost straight away I was back for another battle; another long, cruel battle. It was constant agony and continuous torture, and I knew that I couldn't go on anymore. So eventually I was prescribed the liquid supplements that I had been threatened with. Everyone made it sound like the supplements would be easier, more tolerable – they were to replace my meals when eating was just too difficult. But now I had a choice to make at every meal – eat the food or drink the supplements. I felt like I was being forced to choose between two impossibilities.

Although being prescribed the supplements felt like a huge step backwards, I was determined to fight through it, I was determined to destroy the voice. 'When you keep going down the same path and hitting a wall, sometimes you need to start over and find a different route'. That was what I was told by the doctor. There's no shame in taking a step backwards, there is no shame in starting over – it may have made my journey a little longer, but eventually I knew I would find my path, and my destination would be wonderful.

Although it was agonising, although I felt the anxiety and distress tearing through me like a knife, I fought with every ounce of strength that I had, and for a couple of days I managed to eat. For a couple of days, I found it within myself to commence battle with anorexia once more. I did everything I could to avoid the supplements, and even though it was an immensely hard and gruelling few days, I was finally getting somewhere, I was making progress where I'd failed to make progress before. The thought of the supplements scared me greatly. Liquid calories were one of my greatest fears, yet I knew that it was only a matter of time before I would have to stand up and face the challenge. But just like every other attempt I'd made at moving forwards in recovery, like every other tiny victory that I'd had over the eating disorder, the illness destroyed it. It felt threatened so it pushed me right back to where I'd started. It started telling me that I was doing too well, that I was progressing too quickly. It convinced me that the only way I could prove that I was still suffering, that I still needed help was to resort to the supplements. It was anorexia's sick way of proving how ill I was. It was the eating disorder's twisted way of winning.

Every meal became a test for anorexia, a macabre game to prove how forceful it was. I was no longer allowed to eat food – I was forced to sit in front of plates of fish and chips and burgers and pizzas until I became so distressed, so upset that I was forced to turn to the supplements instead. While every single meal was beating me down into the ground, the eating disorder was thrilled, it was relishing the power. And as its game became bigger, it became stronger, more dominant. It was always the same thing that it was shouting in the back of my mind – I can't do too well, I mustn't succeed, I mustn't put on weight. It was toying with me, squeezing every last drop of fight out of me.

But the supplements proved no easier than the meals. They were just one more opportunity for the eating disorder to have hold over me, to continue its reign of terror. I would bawl and shout to the nurses that it wasn't fair, that none of the other patients had to go through this battle with supplements. I told the staff through my hysterical crying that they were torturing me and

I pleaded with them to stop. But it wasn't them I had to say it to, it was the eating disorder – the illness was the one causing me all of this pain, all of this heartache.

As the weeks went by with no improvement, I was constantly told that I needed to do better, as each week I was completing less and less of my diet. We were constantly looking for another way through but we were rapidly running out of options. I was at the point where my diet consisted only of supplements – the obstacle of food was just too big, too hard to overcome. This way I only had to fight one battle, instead of fighting against both the food and the supplements. Anorexia had full control of my mind and it was not letting go; it was not letting me rest or find peace for a single second. It was in its element and it was using all of the malevolence that it had to destroy me. I prayed for better times, I prayed that this would soon be over, but I knew that recovery depended on me, I knew that I was the only one who could end this.

I would often think back to who I used to be – who I used to be in school and at work, and I felt ashamed. I knew that if my old friends could see me now they wouldn't believe their eyes; the carefree Jade who made everyone laugh, who made everyone smile, was in tears over a 200ml drink. The fearless, confident leader had found her fear – weight gain was her nemesis, food was her enemy. I had become someone else. I had become a victim to anorexia, but I was determined not to remain a victim. I was determined to become a survivor.

To anyone who ever gets confused or doesn't understand why someone with anorexia won't eat,

One of the support workers on the unit once told me this: 'Asking you to eat this bowl of soup is like asking me to eat a bowl full of live spiders. I would be absolutely terrified. I would do anything I can to avoid it.'

That's really stayed with me. It captured exactly how I felt at the time. So remember, if you're ever supporting someone with an eating disorder, think what it would be like to be forced to eat a bowl of live spiders, and then you might get an idea of what they're fighting through, of what they go through each and every day.

*'She took every ounce of strength
left in her bones, and she channelled
it into surviving, into living.'*

BABY STEPS

While I was on the unit I found it harder and harder to find motivation to recover - I lost sight of reality and became so institutionalised that I no longer missed the outside world. Despite all of the challenges I was going through, I felt safe. But there was one thing that I did want to recover for, and that was university.

At the start of my recovery journey, being told I was 'unfit to study' broke my heart. It felt like the end of the world, like all of my dreams had come crashing down around me. Yet at this point, when there were only six months until the start of the new academic year when I could potentially restart again, I saw opportunity. I saw a reality in which I was back studying, back doing what I loved to do. So that became my focus. I had to gain enough weight to get back to university, to be able to physically withstand a demanding hospital placement.

It was terrifying: the thought of having a BMI high enough to go back sent waves of panic crashing through my brain. The idea of having to cope with a placement again when the last one had gone so wrong, when the last one had robbed me of my health and my sanity was awful. But I didn't want to live in a world where the new academic year rolled by, and while everyone else was moving ahead, I was stuck. Stuck in the depths of my eating disorder. Stuck as a patient, when I knew I had what it takes to be a brilliant doctor.

So I began to fight even harder; I began to fight for my future self. I didn't want to look back in a few months and resent myself for not eating a couple of chips or be disappointed in myself for refusing to have a spoonful of yoghurt. I knew I had to suffer the pain and the distress, I knew I had to deal with the fear, and I had to make sure I had no regrets. So although I'd regressed to the point where I was on a completely liquid diet, I fought to eat proper, solid food again. Anorexia was trying to pull me back, to shut me up, but I struggled and I wrestled and I finally stood up and advocated for myself. It was time. I was ready to do this once and for all. This was my mission to conquer.

I knew I was ready, I knew it was time to move from the supplements to proper meals. I was ready to take the leap. It started with a single bite of toast, which seemed like the hardest thing in the universe, but I was moving forwards. Slowly, I was once again taking the first steps to recovery.

From a bite of toast to a spoonful of porridge, to a forkful of scrambled egg. They were baby steps, but they were heading in the right direction. Occasionally I became lost, sometimes I went off course, but the dream of university always got me back on track; it was starting to become my only way of pushing through, my sole reason to recover. But still anorexia held its own. It didn't want me to go back to university, it wanted me to be stuck in this miserable life forever and it was trying its very best to make that happen. It would stop me from eating the batter off my fish, it would stop me from eating the bread with my soup, it would stop me from eating my chocolate bar after lunch and the crisps that came with my sandwich. I was getting stronger, but so was anorexia; while I was fighting harder, anorexia was fighting harder too. There were times when I stood still, progress came to a halt and it was all I could do to hang on, but sometimes just making the effort not to regress is brave and admirable.

Anorexia gave me so many rules surrounding food: always eat the salad or the vegetables first, only have one sugary food item each day, always put your knife and fork down between each mouthful to increase the time of the meal. But throughout this harsh regimen that anorexia imposed upon me, I managed to make myself a new food rule: always leave the table in pain. Never ever walk away from food unless you feel uncomfortable with how much you have eaten. As one of the nurses told me, I had to get comfortable with being uncomfortable. I had to step out of my comfort zone at every chance I had.

At first it was awful, I didn't think I could ever stand to be hurt this much. But throughout my suffering, I managed to learn one of the most important lessons that I've ever learnt from my battles: the feelings won't last. They will build and build; they will crescendo until they are very nearly unbearable, but then they will begin to ebb away. Ever so slowly, the feelings will recede and you will be eventually be free. The anxiety will pass. You will be okay.

I had to remember this through every meal, every snack, every challenge that I faced. It became like a chant: 'the pain won't last, the pain won't last, the pain won't last.' I would whisper it to myself under my breath. I would write it over and over again until it was ingrained in my head. The words became my comfort blanket, the one thing that I could hold onto in times of distress. Those words were what helped me carry on.

My baby steps continued to nudge me forwards, and although each extra bite and each extra spoonful felt like the hardest thing I had ever done, it simply wasn't enough. While I felt like I was achieving extraordinary things, everyone else thought that I wasn't putting enough effort in. While I was ignoring the voice a little bit more each day and pushing forwards, everyone else was telling me I was still giving in to it.

All the while, time was running out and the start of university was creeping ever closer. I knew that the eating disorder was still hanging on, that I was putting my return in jeopardy, but it still wasn't enough to make me complete my diet, to make me eat enough to progress as rapidly as I needed to in order to get back to medical school.

One of the most challenging foods on my meal plan was a small chocolate biscuit bar. Despite the fact that it was lower in calories than many of the other things I was eating, and even though it seemed so small and harmless, to me it was a mountain to climb, a huge fear to conquer. Anyone who knew me before anorexia would tell you that I was a huge chocaholic. I'm not sure there was ever a time I'd say no to chocolate of any sort – it was my ultimate comfort food, my favourite thing in the world. But one thing that

I found out during recovery was that the more I liked the food, the harder it was to eat. The more enjoyment I got from the food, the guiltier anorexia would make me feel for eating it.

I'd been having the chocolate biscuit presented to me for weeks before I finally managed to even unwrap it. The first time it happened my heart was pounding and my hands were shaking, but as soon as I smelt the sweet cocoa wafting towards me I stopped. I knew that if I started to eat it I would never stop. I was scared of losing control. I was scared that if I had a single bite of chocolate after so long avoiding it, I would cave and eat all the chocolate I could get my hands on.

Looking back now, eating the whole bar was the point of having it in my diet plan. If I started and couldn't stop, well that would have been the right thing to do for my recovery, it would have been a hugely positive step forwards. But anorexia would only let me take baby steps; anything more and it would scold me with harsh and despicable words.

So baby steps it was – for a couple of days I just unwrapped the chocolate and did nothing more than enjoy the wonderful smell. If anorexia would have gotten its way I would have stopped there, I would never have pushed myself further, but this time my voice of reason came pushing through and allowed me to have a tiny nibble of the chocolate. I wasn't planning it, I didn't work myself up to this moment, I just took the plunge and went for it. And it was heaven. The chocolate was sweeter than I ever remembered, and it melted on my tongue into a smooth river of deliciousness. My mind instantly took me back to the wonderful memories I had of enjoying food with my family – a Dairy Milk bar before bed, eating Heroes out of the tin at Christmas, cracking open huge eggs at Easter. I felt happy. I was so incredibly proud of myself that the comments that were made about it not being enough, and me giving up too easily simply bounced off me – I knew that I had achieved something huge and NO ONE could take that away from me.

I walked out of the dining room with my head held high and all I wanted was to text my family to tell them that I'd finally eaten chocolate! I knew they'd be so proud of me. But by the time I'd walked the few metres to the lounge the illness had once again woken up and was lecturing me on how ashamed and horrified I should be. I'd given in to the temptation of chocolate. I'd given into my cravings and I was so weak, where had all of my willpower gone?

Well I'll tell you this anorexia, for a moment I was happy. I was proud of myself and you were nowhere to be found. I'd beaten you, and that was where my willpower was. I wasn't weak and I hadn't given in to anything – I'd fought and battled to go against you and I'd succeeded. You were just angry that I'd shown enough strength, courage, and bravery to do something that made me happy. You were angry that just for a moment, I'd won.

SEEDS

As spring time began to fall upon the unit, the occupational therapist helped me to plant some seeds in little flower pots to keep on the windowsill in my bedroom. As they started to bloom I felt immensely proud of both them and myself – I had nurtured these little brown specks of nothingness to become something beautiful. I had devotedly watered them, fed them, and looked after them, and they had rewarded my hard work by doing something incredible – living, growing, thriving. Each morning my first priority would be to rush over to the window to see how much the plants had changed, how much my care had allowed them to bloom.

But it made me stop and think – if I could give all of this love and attention to a plant, why couldn't I do the same for myself? If I was willing to look after a plant so carefully why was I neglecting my body? It opened my eyes to the injustice that I was doing myself – my body deserved to thrive just as much as those seeds, so why was I standing in its way?

To Anorexia,

Three months on, and you're still hanging in there. But not to worry – I'm hanging in there too.

You've chipped away at my life and taken everything I have, well, almost everything. You see, there are some things that are so well protected that you will never get to them. My hope, my determination, my resilience.

It's not just me fighting you anymore – I have an army now. And when I feel too weak to go into battle and I want to wave my flag to surrender, I know that they will pick me up, dust me off, and remind me of all the reasons why I am determined to win this war.

We have weapons that you will never have – bravery, love, courage. Our weapons will ALWAYS win over hatred and hurt, no matter how long you drag this out for, because for them to succeed all they need is for someone to believe. And unfortunately for you, I believe. I believe that I am strong enough to not just conquer you, but to tear you limb from limb with so much force that it's impossible for you to even attempt to pull yourself together again.

I'm not a coward like you are. I will stand and face my battles. I will look you dead in the eye and watch as you crumble. You meanwhile have to hide in your victim's head. You're too scared to show yourself to the world even when you seem to be winning. And that will be your downfall, because cowards can't win over someone who has enough courage to shout and expose your dirty little secrets to the world.

I'm prepared to battle, and I'm planning to win.

PHYSICAL EFFECTS OF ANOREXIA

Although anorexia is a mental illness, it's guaranteed that physical symptoms will plague its sufferers as well. Starving your body does not come without consequences, and often these consequences are brutal, painful, and violent. Eating disorders wreak havoc on the entire body and don't let anything stand in their path.

I suffered horribly with the physical aspects of my illness, however I felt unable to bring the subject up, because anorexia was telling me that it was all self-inflicted. If I told people my body ached all over and I hardly had enough energy to move, surely they'd just tell me to eat more.

If I complained about having no concentration and being unable to focus on anything, wouldn't people just say that I'd brought it on myself? Of course now I realise that none of this is true; this was just one more way that anorexia made me feel invalid and worthless. This was just one more way that anorexia convinced me that I was to blame for everything.

It's a month after I started recovery, and physically I have never felt worse. I'm getting out of my bed and I struggle to sit myself up - my body is desperately eating away at my muscles in an attempt to get energy. My body's even eating away at my heart muscle. I know there's a high risk of me having a heart attack, I know what I'm doing is so dangerous, but surely I won't die – surely that won't happen to me. I manage to get to my feet, but suddenly everything goes black. I don't know where I am, I don't know which way is up, the room is spinning around me.

I manage to clamber into the bathroom and position myself on the toilet, but like the past two weeks, I am dreadfully constipated. Bowel movements aren't possible right now, and even when I do manage one, it's horrendously painful. I know I need to brush my teeth but I don't know if my arms will get through the two minutes; they are so achy. Even if I do manage to brush my teeth, my hair will be a different story. Ponytails are the worst: they ache, they hurt, and my arms simply don't have enough strength in them to tie my hair up.

Getting dressed is the next hurdle. I'm scared to wear any tight-fitting clothing in case I've run out of power to get them off again this evening. So layers it is. Layers and layers of jumpers yet I know I'll still need a hot water bottle and blanket to have any chance of keeping warm. I make my way down the stairs, praying that I won't need to go up them again until bedtime – the muscles in my legs just can't stand it.

I'm curled up on my chair watching TV, but I have no idea what's happening to the characters; I gave up trying to focus on the plot half an hour ago. I pick up my favourite book and try to read instead but I'm too distracted, thinking about food, thinking about what I'm going to eat later on. I need to clear my throat but the muscles in my chest are too weak to allow me to cough. I wonder if I'll end up getting a chest infection or pneumonia. I wonder if my body would be strong enough to be able to fight an infection off.

As the morning draws to a close I'm fighting sleep, fighting to stay awake after last night's insomnia, and the insomnia from every night before. I nap, and when I wake up I wander round the house for a bit just to have something to do, but I don't last long before my chest starts hurting and I find it hard to breathe. So I sit down once more and become anxious about the fact that my life is so sedentary, which leads to me biting and picking at my lips. The blood flows quickly down my chin and they are so sore that no amount of lip balm will be able to cure them.

I mentally prepare myself to eat something, but when I've achieved it my tummy gets big, bloated, and painful. The same with drinking. My digestive system no longer works as it should, and this only serves to make recovery harder and more traumatic. Sometimes I get palpitations after I eat, it feels like my heart is beating out of my chest. A side effect of anxiety? Excitement at treating myself with some new flavours? I really don't know.

Evening rolls around and it's time to have a shower. I dread the day when I have to wash my hair because the physical exertion is nigh on impossible. I run my fingers down my scalp and the hair comes away in clumps. I have to stand and watch it swirl down the drain, inevitably blocking it up little by little. I have the water temperature so hot it feels like bullets striking my skin, but I can't stand to have it any colder. I get out and wrap myself in my towel, before hurrying across the landing to my bedroom. I dread anyone catching me in just my towel because they'll see my body in its true, ugly form.

When I get to my bedroom I seek out the radiator and sit with my back against it. Even though it feels like it's burning, even though it's almost unbearable, it provides temporary relief from the cold. By this time in the day the bones in my bottom are agony from sitting all day. It's too painful to sit, yet too exhausting to stand. I can't win, my body can't win. The eating disorder is ruining me.

As bedtime creeps ever closer I know that the night sweats are coming. As my metabolism learns to cope with the increase in calories I'm taking in, and as my hormones begin to make an appearance again, night sweats become not so much of a problem, just another irritating manifestation of anorexia. I get up in the middle of the night to go to the toilet and my pyjamas are cold and wet through. It's like I've been outside in the rain instead of tucked away safely in my bed. Then I get back underneath the covers and my sheets are soaking. I am repulsed by what my body is doing, I am revolted by this illness, and yet I can't seem to get rid of it. I can't seem to let it go.

I think about myself in 10 years, and the thought of still struggling to eat is abhorrent. I know I need to recover for the sake of my future – if I don't sort this out now I know what problems it can lead to in the long term: infertility, a weakened heart, permanent damage to my brain, osteoporosis. I don't want to get older and suffer because of something that I could have changed in my 20s. It's easier said than done, but sometimes I hate myself for not eating, because I know that I'm putting any future prospects at risk. I need to leave anorexia in the past, not let it control my future.

All of this suffering that my mind is putting my body through is cruel and inhuman, yet somehow I like it, I feel like I deserve it. I relish that ache in my arms and that burning in my legs. The rare times when I get a break from the pain, I long for it to return. I know that this is my penance for starving myself, my punishment for putting my body through Hell. Although I didn't choose to torture myself, although I would stop it if I could, I still have to pay for anorexia's sins. I still have to serve its sentence.

Dear Jade,

Your body is a truly wondrous thing. You are blessed to have a body that has always been healthy and functioning, and that has never let you down.

I know that there are parts of yourself that you don't like – your bumpy nose, your messy hair, your rounded tummy; but they are the least important things about you. You are beautiful and perfect, not despite these things, but because of them.

Look at all of those pictures that you have of yourself before anorexia. Those pictures of you laughing and smiling and shining. The pictures of that strong, confident girl you used to be. When I look at those pictures I see a young lady who was perfect in every way. I don't see all of the things that you hated about the way you looked, I see all of the things that you never realised you had. I see happiness shining out of every pore and a love of life escaping from you. Escaping your body which you were never quite satisfied with, but which is a miracle.

Now look at pictures of yourself with your illness. Look at the tiredness that's replaced the sparkle in your eyes. Look at the effort that shows in your smile compared to the carefree laughter that used to burst from you. See the exhaustion that plagues you now instead of the happiness that you used to emit. You can get all of those things back. They may not be with you right now, but they are out there waiting to join you.

You are beautiful. Your body is so special because it houses a soul that shines. It is your ability to love your imperfections that makes you perfect in every way. Remember to bless your gift with the love it deserves, and be thankful every minute of every single day for the remarkable wonder that you have been given. Your body really is amazing.

A QUICK NOTE
ON PILLS

Just when I thought I was ready to hand in the towel, just when I thought I'd had enough, a new hope was gifted to me. I was given a handful of pills, some of them big and round and pink, some of them narrow and green. With the promise that there was a chance that these could take my pain away, I took them without question, and slowly but surely I began to get a grip on myself again. Okay, things got worse before they got better, but eventually I started to crawl back from wherever anorexia had banished me to, and for just a little while, the screaming in my head dulled ever so slightly. For the briefest moments I could relax without worrying about what I'd just eaten, or what I would be faced with at the next meal. I could find temporary peace in the middle of my distress.

As much as I owe a good part of my recovery to the pills, they weren't the magic cure that I'd hoped for. I still had to push deeper and persevere more than I'd ever done before. I had to fight the fatigue, the brain fog, and the drowsiness that the pills brought and often it became too much effort to stay awake. My life became a cycle of 'eat, sleep, repeat', and I spent my days either at the dinner table or unable to move off the sofa. Even when I was awake I was so drowsy that my eyes couldn't focus and I hardly had enough strength to hold up my own head. My anxiety improved, but at a huge cost. After all the work I was putting into eating, the rest of my energy was spent on trying to stay awake. However, at times I welcomed the nothingness. I welcomed a chance to get through the day without having anorexia attack my mind. The sweet relief of falling asleep for hours, of having some time blissfully unaware of the pain was amazing. But I was confused, I was disorientated, and I wasn't present. I wasn't living, but the choice between being disconnected from my body and having the voice scream at me every minute of every day was easy – I took the pills.

I was jealous of the other patients who got through recovery without medication. Perhaps it just didn't work for them, or perhaps they chose not to become detached from reality like I did. I know that needing medication to function doesn't make me weak, and I know that it doesn't define the severity of my eating disorder. Even now, over a year later, I look at the pills in my hand every morning and night and wish that I didn't have to take them. I consider throwing them in the bin, saving myself from the horrendous feelings that I know will befall me in a couple of hours, but every time I pick up the water and I swallow them. I swallow them knowing that I'm fighting, and knowing that one day I will be able to function just perfectly without any help.

'The stars aligned, and her spirit came alive.'

GAINING WEIGHT

Recovery doesn't happen overnight. If it did there would be no need for specialist eating disorder hospitals. For me, a huge part of recovery involved gaining back the weight that I had lost through my self-imposed starvation, and I was absolutely petrified. I wish more than anything there was a pill to stop people being scared of weight gain. I wish there was a drip that you could be put on that suddenly took away the voice in your head. It doesn't seem fair that people with anorexia have to work so damn hard to recover, when their illness has already beaten them to the ground. It's not fair that innocent people have to give up their lives and their livelihoods to fight off something which never should have put them through hell in the first place.

A few months into my admission to the specialist eating disorder unit, I still hadn't made any significant progress. I'd endured the supplements, I'd put up with the agonising anxiety of trying to eat solid foods again, but I'd ended up falling right back to where I'd started. I'd exhausted just about every plan the nurses could think of to help me, and I was worried that I'd become a hopeless case that everyone would eventually give up on.

Every week I was told that I wasn't doing well enough. Every week I was terrified of stepping on the scales because although I wanted to get to a point where I could get discharged and go home, the thought of weight gain was still terrifying. I don't have an explanation as to why weight gain was so scary. I don't really understand it myself – I know the fear is irrational but that doesn't stop it from haunting me, from being with me every minute of every day. I felt that if I gained weight my world would end. I felt like weight gain would be a disaster, a disaster I wouldn't be able to live through.

While I was an inpatient I got weighed first thing every Tuesday morning. Every Monday night I would obsessively check my tummy to make sure it didn't feel bigger and more bloated than usual. I would read my book for as long as I could to make myself tired, because I knew the chances of well-needed sleep that night were slim; I knew my dreams would be constantly interrupted by anxiety. Every Tuesday morning I would wake up hours before I needed to, and when the drowsiness passed and I remembered that I had to be weighed that morning, my heart would instantly start trying to beat out of my chest with fright. I frantically tried to find something to distract me, but I still ended up watching the clock, watching the minutes tick away until I could get this over and done with.

At 7am I would cut my finger nails, go to the toilet as many times as I could, shave myself; anything to get rid of what I perceived as extra weight. I believed that long fingernails or slightly more body hair would make me appear heavier. I would never put any hand cream on the night before or spray any deodorant until after I'd been weighed, because surely the cream and deodorant would add weight to me. I knew it was crazy, I knew that doing all of these things was insane, but somehow they allowed my mind to rest easy. They allowed the eating disorder to be happy with me for about five minutes every week.

I'd change into my night dress that I got weighed in and make my way downstairs with shaking legs and short, panicked breaths. I never wore my glasses or my watch. I even took my hair tie out so as not to add any extra weight. I'd take a deep breath, close my eyes, and step up to the scales, ready to find out my fate. If I breathe in will the number be higher, or am I better to breathe out? What if I'm inadvertently affecting the reading? But then I hear the beep of the machine and I know that I can't change anything now.

I slowly open my eyes with dread. The number that I see will determine how my week will go. This number will be my focus for the next seven days until I get weighed again. I am living for these few minutes each week when I get to see what my weight has done. Every bite of food or sip of water that I take, I'm thinking about how it will affect that number. When I've seen the display I take off back upstairs to my bedroom, and whatever the result I will probably cry. Either crying with relief or crying with fear. How can a number make me feel like this? How can so much in my life depend on such a small aspect of who I am?

Two years on, and I still do all of those mad things before I'm weighed. I always choose my lightest clothes to wear, I still make sure my nails are cut as short as possible. Maybe I just do them out of habit, or maybe somewhere inside me, I still believe that not doing these things will make me appear heavier on the scales. I try to tell myself that all of these things are crazy, that by doing this I'm pushing myself deeper into the eating disorder, but I'm loathed to stop. I know that if I stop my anxiety will become all-consuming. I know that if I stop I will have to endure even more distress and fear than I'm already fighting against. I'm desperately clinging on to these behaviours but they are strengthening the eating disorder. I know I have to let them go but I am terrified.

Some people are scared of snakes, some people are scared of heights. I am scared of gaining weight. I'm scared of my BMI increasing, and of the number on the scales getting bigger. The fear is so irrational, yet there's nothing that I can do to make it better. There's nothing that will stop me from being scared. I know that to recover I need to gain weight, I know that I don't want to suffer like this for the rest of my life, but sometimes it just feels too hard. I don't see food, I see calories, I see weight gain. I don't see something that's going to taste nice and satisfy me, I see something which will push up the dreaded number, which will make my thighs bigger and my face chubbier.

Anorexia made me believe so many crazy things about weight gain:

- If I put on lipgloss and accidentally ingested any of it I would gain weight
- If I swallowed toothpaste it would make

me gain weight
- If I went outside in the rain and got even a little bit wet my weight would go up because my body would soak up the water like a sponge
- Taking tablets for indigestion would make me gain weight

I never ever allowed myself to drink before I was weighed, sometimes I even went more than 18 hours without fluids, because I was so scared of what the water would do to the scales.

But the thing with gaining weight is, you will always regain something else alongside it which the eating disorder caused you to lose. As well as gaining body mass, you will regain a life, you will regain friends who you once lost, and you will regain the ability to concentrate and do things you enjoy. You will regain the freedom that's been torn away from you, and you will regain your personality. You will be able to be happy again, your body will no longer ache with every movement, and you will be able to sleep again.

Although gaining weight seemed like the worst thing that could possibly happen to me, I came to realise that it was a necessity. It didn't make it any easier, and it didn't stop me crying, but every time the scales showed a number which I didn't like, I told myself that it was just my life returning. It was the only way I was going to get my freedom back.

Dear Jade,

To be brave is to feel the fear and trepidation, to become weak at the knees and have your hands shake, to feel the butterflies in your tummy and the pounding of your heart, and do what scares you anyway. Bravery isn't the absence of fear or never feeling scared, bravery is being the most scared you've ever been in your life yet still managing to push through to the other side of the rainbow. Bravery doesn't have to be special, it doesn't have to be magnificent, in fact it won't feel amazing at all. It will feel hard and exhausting. It will feel impossible and out of reach.

But know that when all you see is darkness and misery, everyone else is seeing your light. When all you see is yourself getting out of bed, everyone else sees your courage to carry on and continue fighting. When all you see is yourself living, everyone else sees you refusing to give up.

Things that make you brave:

- *You are here, living and breathing*
- *You get out of bed every day, no matter how fed up, and how exhausted you are*
- *You have felt like giving up so many times, but you're still fighting*
- *You have a complete breakdown and cry hysterically, then you get back up and carry on*
- *You are moving forward, even though you*

can't see the final destination

- *You keep facing the same battles, with confidence that one time you will win*

- *You do things that make you feel uncomfortable, and then do them again and again*

- *You find it in yourself to be kind and thoughtful towards other people fighting battles, when you're busy fighting battles of your own*

- *You refuse to let life break you, however much it tries*

- *You stand up each and every day with your head held high, and you never ever let anything stand in your way*

MOVING FORWARDS

As time in the inpatient unit flew by, it looked like I was finally beginning to make some good progress. To the outside world, I was taking more risks, I was choosing to be brave, and it seemed like I was trying to defy the eating disorder at every turn. Things were certainly starting to get better, but they were still far from perfect.

While the eating disorder would allow me to go out and buy a sandwich for my lunch, it was anorexia who dictated what filling I had. While the voice finally quietened down when I ate my chocolate bar, it always made me choose the one with the least calories, even though there were only 10 calories difference. While anorexia was permitting me to eat more and more each day, I still wasn't in control. I was still a slave to the eating disorder.

I would go out to the shop to buy my own snack, and I could spend what felt like forever examining the calorie count on all of the options. I knew what I wanted, and I knew what the eating disorder wanted, yet I also knew that anorexia would still always win. I was eating to get discharged. I was eating to make my life easier and stop staff from pushing me to my limits. I was eating to go home, to get back to university - that was my only motivation, my only reason to gain weight, to recover.

But whatever my reason, I was eating. I was trying so hard to put my fears behind me and move on with my life. I wasn't always successful, but when I was, I knew that I was just one step closer to a life without the eating disorder.

I was gaining weight, and I was completing more of my diet, but my mind was still suffering. There were still battles wreaking havoc on my brain, but now I could fight them with the knowledge that they would end, and I had a chance of winning. I was still putting up with the pain and anxiety of eating proper meals, but now I knew that the negative feelings would eventually fade. The storm was still ongoing, but I was powering through it. I was learning to dance in the rain.

At every single meal I pushed myself further than I'd ever been before. I pushed myself so far out of my comfort zone, I could no longer see where it ended. Sometimes it was a few grains of rice, and sometimes it was several chips, but every single time I sat down to eat, I ate more than last time. Every single time I got up from the dining table I made sure I felt the pain and the torment in my mind, because that was how I knew that I was properly beating this thing. It didn't matter if I was still full from the previous meal, it didn't even matter if I'd just got weighed and had a huge gain – I knew the most important thing for me to do was to keep moving forwards and improve little by little.

It was unbearably difficult and excruciatingly slow, and sometimes I wondered if I would ever manage to eat 'normally' again. But I held onto hope and refused to give up. There were days when I didn't think I could fight any longer, and there were days when I cried alone for hours in my bedroom because I thought that there was no way forward. But on every one of these days I did the exact same thing: I rested, I forgave myself, and I knew that I wouldn't feel like that forever. I went to sleep content with the knowledge that I could try again in the morning.

It was a long road, and some days I walked further than others, but I was learning so much along the way. Through all of my therapy, I was finally starting to accept that not only was my illness real, it was valid and I deserved treatment, no matter how long it had lasted for or how much I restricted my intake at my worst. I was learning that I was allowed to eat and I was allowed to nourish my body, and it wasn't greedy or selfish to do so. I was learning not to be so hard on myself, and to fully respect my body and my mind. Most importantly, I was learning to recognise the tricks that anorexia was using against me to keep me trapped in the eating disorder, and I was working so extremely hard to defeat it.

Despite all of my agonising efforts, my dreams of returning to university almost a year after I'd been forced to take a leave of absence slowly ground to a halt. I think I'd known for some time that I wasn't ready for the huge commitment of becoming a medical student again, but still the hope burned strong inside me, giving me purpose and strength to move forwards in treatment. So when the dreaded news that I still wasn't fit to return to study came, I crumbled. My courage wavered and I felt lost. I'd lost the one motivation that I had to eat, which was helping me to recover despite all of the pain and the screaming going on inside my head. Despite all of the guilt and self-loathing, eating was going to be so worth it to go back to university; what was I supposed to do now? Now that my future was so uncertain and messy?

But through the disappointment I realised that somewhere along the way I had found another reason to recover. I was recovering to regain every single thing that anorexia had stolen from me – my independence, my happiness, and most of all my life. My wonderful little life which may not have been perfect, but in which I was happy and free. My life which allowed me to follow my dreams and become whoever I wanted to be.

So I carried on moving forwards. The news about university was just one more hurdle to jump along the track of my recovery, just one more thing I had to overcome to continue on my path. I ate, and I slept, and then I ate some more. Somehow I found it within myself to take great leaps towards recovery. With the greatest courage and the most incredible bravery, I began to eat everything that was put in front of me. I just wanted to get out of the unit and go home, I wanted to get back to being who I was born to be. It was painful, at times it was agonising, but I dealt with the pain because I knew that it was leading to somewhere brilliant.

I was tired. I was tired of fighting myself, and I was tired of fighting everyone around me. I longed for just one easy day – one day when

I could take time off from having an eating disorder. But anorexia is a full-time job. In fact it's more than just a full-time job, it's with you every morning, every afternoon, every evening, and every night. It doesn't release you from its clutches just because it's your birthday or Christmas, and it doesn't care if you've got a big celebration meal to go out for, it just uses these things to make you feel even more guilty, even more depressed about the fact that you can't join in and the fact that you're 'ruining' the day for everyone else. It's constant. It's exhausting.

But the further I got into recovery, and the more of these special occasions I 'ruined', the more I realised that you make memories every single day, and in the grand scheme of things those days mean nothing, they're just arbitrary dates on a calendar with no real meaning. In ten years time I know I won't look back and remember not eating Christmas dinner for one year, I will remember the time when I was happy and healthy and we ate turkey in August, just because I wanted to. I won't remember my exact birthday where I didn't allow myself to have any cake, but I will remember 6 months later when I was in a much better place and I ate the most delicious slice of chocolate cake in the world. I won't remember missing out on a takeaway for someone's birthday, but I will remember ordering a pizza, regardless of what day it was because that's what I fancied.

I'm not saying that these days aren't important, I'm just saying that they can be celebrated at any time of year, when I'm ready, and when I can enjoy them with no limitations. I was lucky to know that my family cared more about my wellbeing than having a 'normal' Christmas, and I was lucky to know that they understood the times when joining in was too much for me. But I swear I will make up for those missed opportunities, those missed memories. I will eat all of the cake and all of the turkey and the stuffing that I missed out on, and I will do it with joy and freedom and delight. I will do it without anorexia.

Dear Jade,

Look at you. Look how far you've come. Remember how you felt a few months ago – like there was no hope, like you'd never see the light again, and think about how much courage it took to get to where you are now. Things that would have terrified you before are now not only easier, but almost enjoyable. Things that you never thought you could do, you've smashed the hell out of them. Just keep going because I am SO proud of you, and I know you can get to where you want to be.

There's still a long way to travel, but when the destination is as amazing as this, it doesn't matter about the journey. It doesn't matter about all the times you slipped up; you'll learn from them. It doesn't matter that the path was messy and winding; a straight path is just plain boring. It doesn't matter that you went through so much pain to get here, because the path leads home. And once you are home, you can spread your wings and fly.

ANOREXIA'S PURPOSE

Anorexia made me feel strong, when in every other aspect of my life I felt weak. It made me feel worthy, when I'd convinced myself that I was worthless. Anorexia gave me a sense of achievement when I was desperately searching for a reason to feel good about myself. It served a purpose, but I don't want it to burden me anymore. My starved body felt numb, even when I should have been fighting off the biggest emotions. The illness gave me a reason to rest and rehabilitate when I felt like I didn't deserve to take a break. My mind felt unbreakable and undefeatable, yet my body was weak and failing.

What purpose did Anorexia serve for me? Maybe I wanted to feel more in control of my life. Maybe I needed a way to cope with the uncertainty of the future. For me, food was the answer to all of my problems. It was one thing in my life that I could control, that I could take charge of.

Different people use food in different ways to control their emotions. Some people overeat, some people undereat, there are so many different behaviours that can bring someone calmness during their storm. I 'chose' to undereat. I put chose in quotation marks because even though I thought I was making my own choices, I most certainly was not.

While I was spending my days completing my medical school placement, while I was trying my best to become a good doctor, something had grabbed hold of me when I wasn't looking. I began to find ways of making myself feel better, of finding comfort when I needed it the most. If I felt like I hadn't achieved much on a particular day, I would go home and restrict my food intake, then wait until the monster in my head congratulated me for resisting the temptation of more food. If I had made a mistake on placement and felt like I was unworthy to be a medical student, the monster would force me to wait longer and longer until my stomach was empty and I had hunger pains, and then tell me that I was strong and I had punished myself for what had happened that day.

I was just trying to find peace in the chaos erupting all around me. I was just trying to find calmness during my storm.

I believed that I was proving to everyone how strong I was, how powerful I was. But I wasn't strong for denying myself food, I was strong for exposing the illness. Eating less didn't make me any more or less worthy than I already was – I know now that I'm always worthy of happiness and content. Starving myself wasn't an achievement, but beginning to eat again was. Beginning to eat again was my biggest ever achievement.

I know now that I'm allowed to take breaks to look after myself, and I'm allowed to admit I need help. I'm allowed to have bad days where I don't get out of bed, but I'm also allowed to have bloody brilliant days where I thrive and don't give a care in the world.

Anorexia acts like it's in control, but I know that only I can change my own destiny. Anorexia feels big and overwhelming, but I know that my mind can be bigger, and my thoughts can be more resilient. I know that I can start any time I want, and I know that I can change my life. I know that with hard work and dedication, I can save myself from this torture, from this torment.

CHAIR REST

After spending months as an inpatient and missing my home so deeply and intensely, I began to see change within myself. Some changes were for the better, some for the worse. I was happier and more confident, I became less anxious and I could finally laugh again. But at the same time the eating disorder had become even more a part of my life than it was before. Every waking minute was spent thinking about anorexia, because I was surrounded by people with the illness. Every day it became more a part of who I was, and I had less and less respite from it.

When I was first diagnosed with anorexia, my body was too compromised to function properly. My heart was so weak, and my muscles were constantly under strain; just standing up required huge amounts of effort. The doctors forbade me from all types of exercise, from walking around a shop to standing in a queue – it was simply too dangerous, I simply didn't have enough energy in me. When I was admitted to the inpatient unit I was faced with the same rules, I wasn't even allowed to take the stairs to my bedroom until I hit a certain BMI. It was called 'chair rest'. I watched longingly as the other patients would go out for walks in the park and do yoga classes, wishing that I could do the same, getting increasingly frustrated as I missed out on more and more activities. It was yet another reason to be furious at anorexia, just another reason to recover.

Every time I put weight on I tried to feel better by telling myself that I was one step closer to getting off chair rest, one step closer to gaining just a tiny glimmer of freedom in this life of restrictions. It was the only thing I focused on because it was the only good thing I could think of to come from gaining weight. Every time the eating disorder told me not to eat the burger or the pizza, I would retaliate with the fact that I longed to have more freedom, that I longed to reach the stage where my body wasn't too fragile to allow me to stand up. The closer I got to being able to come off chair rest, the more I started envisioning everything that I would be able to do when the time came. I saw a glimpse of light ahead, and I was striving to reach it.

The day that I was finally allowed off chair rest I felt the change before it was confirmed - I somehow knew that the moment had come at last. I went downstairs to get weighed like every other Tuesday, but this week a tiny bit of the anxiety had been replaced with hope. I kept telling myself that it didn't matter how much weight I'd put on, as long as it was enough to get me above that long-awaited BMI. I repeated and repeated this little reassurance until I tricked my mind into believing it to be true. As I stepped on the scales and looked over at my new weight, this new weight which would allow me a small taste of freedom, the anxiety still rushed around my body. The terror that I felt at gaining weight still gripped me, but I was able to tell myself that it was all worth it – all of the previous weeks of suffering and torment had led up to today. The day when I knocked down another barrier on my path to recovery.

I knew that a world of possibilities had just opened up to me. The thought of having such freedom, the thought of being able to go out by myself for the first time in months petrified me, but it was a good kind of scared. It was a brilliant kind of scared. However anorexia was furious – how dare I meet this huge milestone? How dare I make progress in my quest to be rid of it? While everyone was congratulating me on my achievement, telling me how well I'd done, I was willing them to stop talking, to stop provoking the eating disorder even further. It resented the praise, it despised the positivity that was surrounding me. While I got the phrase 'well done' raining down on me from all directions, all I wanted was a shield to stop the agony that it was causing me. I'd been waiting for this moment for so long, I had worked so hard to get here, I should have been delighted. But I quickly fell into a pit of despair.

I was allowed to go off the unit for walks, but they weren't fun; they were driven by anorexia. I would walk as far as I possibly could every day in a bid to stop gaining weight. I would go up and down the stairs every time I could think of a plausible excuse to burn just a few more calories. I once again became obsessed with how much exercise I was doing – I was constantly on edge, always feeling the need to move. Anorexia took full advantage of my new freedom; it told me that I was lazy and disgusting if I wasn't being active. Now that I was allowed to do these things, I had no excuse.

My first week in a new phase of recovery was the hardest week I'd been through for a long time. I started restricting again, more than I had for quite some time. All that was running through my head was that I absolutely HAD to lose weight this week. I had no other option. I was convinced that if I weighed more next time I stepped on the scales it would be the end of the world. It would be impossible for me to carry on living.

All week my mind tortured me. Every meal was a battle between me and the eating disorder, it was constantly telling me that I was recovering too quickly, that I was putting weight on too quickly. In this absurd world of eating disorders, somehow having the power to be able to walk again equalled full recovery. Somehow having permission to use a set of stairs instead of a lift symbolised a full return to health. I'd become so used to being so poorly, that when I began to feel remotely better, when I began to feel a little less tired, a little less achy, I managed to convince myself that I was recovered. I thought that despite still being in hospital, despite still being horrified every time I put on a tiny bit of weight, the war was over. But nothing could have been further from the truth – I was still severely ill. I still had hundreds more terrible and harrowing battles to fight.

The following week I lost weight and found the privileges that I'd worked so hard to gain ripped away from me. Although it was a step back, I felt calmer, safer. I didn't realise it at the time, but now I know that by allowing my eating disorder to be content and secure, by staying well within my comfort zone, I not only delayed my recovery, I fell backwards into a trap which would take insane amounts of work to escape. I had not only allowed anorexia to become more indestructible, I had allowed myself to become more fragile and vulnerable once again.

The new rein of anorexia lasted a further three weeks. Another three weeks until I was in a position to fight again to take the next steps in recovery. I was allowed back off chair rest, and I was prepared for what was coming this time. I was prepared for the hate, and the fury, and the intensity of what the eating disorder was going to throw at me. I knew that I couldn't allow myself to fall again, so I stood and fought like a warrior. Yes, the eating disorder was still shouting at me, and yes, it was giving me a million reasons not to eat, but I put all of my effort into disobeying it. I swore I would never again allow anorexia's thoughts to poison my brain, to taint my mind. I swore this would be the end of the loathing and the start of my victory.

Dear Jade,

You are beautiful because you're you. You stand out from the crowd because you work so hard and you are so talented. You are extraordinary as you are. You don't need to change anything about yourself to influence how other people think about you.

Don't let other peoples' opinions get under your skin. You are NOT important to them and in years to come you won't even remember their name. The people who surround you may feel important right now but believe it or not, people come and go.

The ones that matter are family. Whether that's blood-relations or the type of family you can choose. Making the most of the time you spend with them is what will bring you happiness. Making them proud will bring you joy. Just being in their company will soothe your heart and soul.

There will always be someone better than you, smarter than you, more accomplished than you. And that's okay. You are unique and no one possesses the same qualities you do. Yes, you need to work hard in life, and yes, you need to throw yourself into everything you do. But you don't need to sacrifice other aspects of your life to be the best. As long as you're happy and you're utilising your full potential, you don't need to do anything more.

You are perfect, and your life is pretty damn

awesome. Embrace it.

CHOICES

Throughout my recovery, the voice spent a lot of time telling me what was 'right' and what was 'wrong'. The 'right' order to eat things. The 'right' way to cut my toast. The 'right' cereal to have. Anorexia made every little decision about food or eating feel like an ultimatum, it made it feel like my whole future was dependent on what flavour yoghurt I chose.

The eating disorder was constantly threatening me, warning me against making the 'wrong' decision. If I chose to eat the 'wrong' half of my sandwich first, if I chose the 'wrong' banana to eat, I had been convinced that terrible things would happen. I was convinced that I wouldn't be safe, I wouldn't be loved.

My life revolved around these decisions. Every meal was a test – would I succeed and do what was 'right', or would I fail and do something that anorexia deemed to be 'wrong'? It made me eat food in size order – small to large. If two pieces of food were the same size the decision over which to eat first would feel impossible. It made me eat my pieces of toast from the one with the least marmite first, to the one with the most marmite last. But what if the piece with the least marmite was the biggest? What was I supposed to do then? Go from small to large, or go from least marmite to most marmite?

It also convinced me that there were 'right' and 'wrong' choices when I was deciding what to eat. Do I have weetabix or do I have porridge? Do I have a cheese sandwich or an egg sandwich? Usually the answer was clear – whatever had the least calories. But I also had to make sure that I wasn't 'wasting' calories on foods I didn't like, or that I wasn't in the mood for. My anxiety peaked every time I tried a new food, because if it wasn't perfect, if I didn't love it, I felt like the calories that I'd consumed from that food were 'wasted'.

Most of the time I managed to keep the voice happy, but those few wrong decisions that I made felt like the end of the world. With each wrong decision came a whirlwind of fury, a taste of anorexia's wrath. With each wrong decision came even more suffering, and even more pain.

I still play by these crazy rules years later. I

still feel compelled to eat my strawberries from smallest to largest, I still feel obliged to cut my sandwich so that one piece is clearly bigger than the other, just so that I have no doubt which to eat first. Each time I feel the need to do these rituals I try to stop myself, I try to talk myself out of it, but the anxiety and the discomfort are too intense. I tell myself that doing these things is okay – surely the most important thing is actually eating the food, no matter what order I do it in. But on the other hand I know that this seemingly insignificant compulsion has the potential to escalate into the eating disorder taking full control again.

'Through the darkness came a shining beacon of hope. A force so strong that she felt it with every fibre of her being, and she believed in it with everything she had.'

HOME LEAVE

Seven months into my inpatient stay, I was faced with some of the biggest challenges I would encounter while I was on the unit. Challenges that had the power to either launch me forward in recovery, or stubbornly hold me back. As I became more accustomed to being off chair rest, my independence slowly started crawling back to me, but now my mind was full of conflict between myself and the eating disorder. Conflict over whether I should go for a walk in the park or let my body rest. Conflict over whether I should stand up in order to burn just a few more calories while I was waiting for my medications; or whether I should sit down, like my body was begging me to do. These decisions may not seem huge, but to me they were everything. They were the difference between allowing the eating disorder to retain that tiny bit of control, or breaking free from the illness for just a few minutes each day. It was agonisingly hard to rebel against anorexia, and each decision was laced with guilt. But sometimes, I won. Sometimes, for just a little while, I was able to triumph against the monster in my head.

As time went on I accepted that I was progressing through recovery and even though I still had a lot of awful days, a few better days began to become interspersed with them. On these better days I would joke with the staff, I would laugh with the other patients, and I would engage in conversation at the dining table – three simple things which I thought anorexia had stolen from me forever. As spring turned to summer and the world became a little bit brighter, I was confronted with my next challenge to conquer - home leave.

Leaving the unit behind me and being allowed to go home for a couple of days was one of the most exciting, yet one of the most nerve-wracking things that I experienced during my recovery. Although I was making substantial progress as an inpatient, the safety and support wouldn't be with me forever. I had to get used to eating by myself, eating when nobody was pushing me forward to face my fears. I had to get used to fighting the voice in my head when no one from the unit was there to drown out the noise.

My turn for leave came just at the right time -

just when I thought I couldn't bear it any longer on the unit with nothing to look forward to, nothing to keep me going; just as I began feeling rather downcast and fed up with the monotony of what my life had become. I missed so many things about being home – I missed sitting in my favourite chair and watching quiz shows with my family. I missed sleeping in my own bed, in the familiar security of my bedroom. I missed being surrounded by people who made me feel warm and comfortable, who made it known that they would never ever leave me, no matter how horrendous the storm that I was battling through became.

But home leave came with a million choices. A million different decisions which all had to be right, which all had to be perfect. I had the freedom to decide, for the first time since I'd been admitted to hospital all of those months ago, what I wanted to eat for each meal. I had the freedom to do as much physical exercise as I wanted, without being limited to half an hour in the park. But with that freedom came intense pressure. Pressure from the eating disorder not to put on weight. Pressure from myself to continue progressing in recovery.

In the days before I went home, I spent hours trying to put together the perfect meal plan. Now that anorexia was allowing me to eat more, challenge different foods, and worry less about calorie counting, I thought that it would be easy, I thought that my mind would allow me to eat whatever I wanted. But I soon realised that I was wrong. My mind was determined to ruin this for me, to take this opportunity and use it to halt my progress in its tracks. It convinced me that the 'right' choice was the one with the least possible number of calories, the 'right' choice was to lose weight. And I believed the voice. All of the hard work I'd done to defy it left me, and I once again took to the internet, comparing the calories of different sandwich fillings and different snack options. The eating disorder was compelling me to create the perfect meal plan which would set me back in recovery. It was a despicable mission set by anorexia. A mission designed to torment me and beat me down.

I was too ashamed to tell anyone. After doing so well in the weeks leading up to my leave, I was ashamed to admit that I was once again letting anorexia get to me. I was overwhelmed and I was tired. Tired of fighting against myself all of the time. But the eating disorder was so proud, and it was that pride that I cherished and held on to.

My anxiety hit an all-time high as my Dad drove me home. I knew that I'd become a different person since I last saw my family, and I had no idea how they expected me to be now. Would they be disgusted at how much I ate? Would they be ashamed of me? Would they still accept me for who I had become? Meanwhile the eating disorder was clinging on tight, taking advantage of my fears; my fears of facing it alone for the first time in months. I was getting more used to fighting and disobeying the voice on the unit, but I wasn't sure if I possessed enough courage yet to do it at home as well.

The house felt comfortable yet unnerving, familiar yet strange. The sights, the smells, everything that I'd never noticed before came rushing at me, reminding me of where I truly belonged. I didn't belong in this cruel world of eating disorders - I was worth so much more than that. But still I soldiered on, following anorexia's guide every step of the way. Every meal was a chance to restrict my food intake, every snack a chance to cut calories. My Mum and I would go on beautiful countryside walks and all I could think about was how many steps I was doing, whether I was doing more or less than my daily route around the park near the inpatient unit.

At first I'd thought that home leave would be a break from constantly being surrounded by thoughts of anorexia, but it turned out to be the opposite – the voice was louder and more persistent than ever. I'd thought that by listening to the voice, by doing what it wanted of me, my anxiety would diminish; but it remained as strong and as forceful as ever before.

But I knew that this wasn't the end of the road - although my meal plan was far from ideal, I managed to stick to it, which I saw as an achievement. Although my anxiety was high, I managed to relax and enjoy the mundaneness of everyday life, which I saw as a positive in a muddle of negatives. I knew that despite my illness, I was lucky. I was lucky enough to be able to try going home again the following week, and each week after that. I was lucky enough to be able to go easy on myself instead of feeling guilty about succumbing once again to the eating disorder. I was lucky enough to be given another chance to prove to myself, and everyone around me that I was strong enough to beat this. That I was brave enough to keep fighting.

To Anorexia,

I can see a tiny spark of light ahead. I am Jade, and I am doing this for me. You'll say that I'm selfish and force horrendous feelings of guilt onto me, but I can brush them off now because I know that they're all lies. You'll tell me that people will think that I'm weak, a failure, if I eat, but I don't care anymore. Throw everything at me – hate, terror, fear. I am ready. I am ready to conquer every challenge and endure every storm.

You keep saying that I'm doing too well, but guess what? There's no such thing. When my tummy hurts from eating so much and I feel fat and greedy, I know that it's you feeling those things, and I feel proud for beating you. When I put on weight and you tell me that I'm a horrible person, that I am despicable and disgusting, I feel excited because I'm one step closer to leaving you behind.

You want me to be as ill as possible for as long as possible. You get a kick out of ruining my recovery and you're thrilled at the thought of me being the victim. You tell me that I'm nothing without you; that I won't be loved, won't be appreciated without you hanging on to me. But you're wrong - without you I am free to be whoever I want to be. I am free to grow and flourish.

For a while the lines separating us were blurred – we merged into one another. But now I can separate us. I can see you clearly for what you are: a thief, stealing away the lives of innocent people. A captor, holding its victims down in chains. A monster, preying on those who deserve to be happy and free.

You have lied to me for so long and convinced me that you were my friend. You have deceived me and misled me. You have beaten me and broken me. But not anymore; now I can see the truth.

The truth is, I am so much stronger than you. I am so much braver than you, and I will win. I refuse to play your silly games any longer - I know who I am now, and you can never, ever take that away from me.

SAMMY

Being an inpatient is weird. Anorexia forces you to compete with all of these other people with the same illness, yet you end up making friends. You end up supporting each other. You end up being closer to some of these people than your own family. In that moment you understand each other, in fact it's like everyone else in the world is speaking a new language, and you and your fellow patients are the only ones who still understand each other.

I learnt so much from the other patients on the unit, and I owe some of them equal recognition as the staff for playing a part in my recovery. When I had thoughts running around my head that were so crazy that I was too embarrassed to voice them to a nurse, I would tell another patient and get reassurance that it was normal – they'd suffered the same thing. When I felt fat and bloated and sick, I knew I could let my frustrations out to another patient and hear understanding, instead of people trying to rationalise it, trying to pretend like they understood.

We watched films together, we looked at clothes online together, we chatted together about anything and everything. We were closer than sisters, yet to anorexia we were enemies, competing in this sick game that the illness made us play. One minute we could be gossiping about the latest news, and the next I would have to watch as a close friend broke down over half a plate of fries. One minute we would be laughing and telling jokes to each other, and the next I would witness the tears streaming down their face as they went through one of the worst moments of their life. Being forced into each others' company when everyone was at their worst, we had no choice but to bond, we had no choice but to become each others' closest confidants and biggest champions. We hugged each other when we cried, and we cheered for each other when we accomplished something great. We were an army.

Saying this, being an inpatient was incredibly hard at times. I saw and heard things that I don't think I'll ever forget. I heard a young, scared teenager screaming through the night while she was sectioned under the Mental Health Act and forced to consume calories. I heard one of my new friends sobbing that life was too hard and she didn't want to live anymore. I heard the patient in the room next to me banging her head on the wall so hard she had to get taken to A&E. There were emergency alarms going off when people had tried to commit suicide. There were people wrapped in bandages like mummies from where they had harmed themselves. There were people breaking and falling to pieces all over the place, yet I had to stay strong. I couldn't let my recovery be dictated by other people.

It was hard to eat a meal with everything that was going on in my head, but it was even harder when all around me people were beside themselves with pain and hurt. The girl who sat next to me would cry into her mashed potato and I had no power to stop it; all I wanted in that very moment, more than I wanted my own hurt to go away, was to give her some comfort and stop her distress. The teenager a couple of tables away would be shaking with fear over her sausages and gravy, yet I couldn't bring her any relief. I couldn't fix any of them, just like I couldn't fix myself.

I made a lot of wonderful and inspiring friends, but one of the best friends I made during inpatient treatment was a girl named Sammy. She was ten years older than me, and had been suffering with anorexia for years, a lot longer than I had, but still we bonded and she was one of the most kind, caring, and supportive people I've ever met. She had been admitted one week before me, so we were on similar treatment paths – our portion sizes were increased together, we were on chair rest together, we sat together in the dining room. We truly were in this together – every challenge that we faced, we faced together. We would sit next to each other in the lounge and even nap on adjacent sofas during the day. We bonded through our similarities, but in the end it was our differences that made me respect her and envy her more than anyone I'd ever met.

At the start I didn't want to recover; I wanted to eat less and less, and I wanted to continue losing weight. Even when I was admitted to hospital, even when I first went to the specialist unit, I still wasn't finished with the eating disorder, I didn't feel ill enough to begin recovering. And I thought that was how I was supposed to be, I thought that's how people expected me to feel. But Sammy was different: she owned her recovery. She ate everything on her plate and she did it with determination and strength. She cried, she wanted to give up, and some days she didn't even feel like getting out of bed; but still she showed up, she cared for me as well as for herself, and she showed her eating disorder who was boss. Sammy gave me faith. She showed me that I was allowed to go against the illness, and she held my hand as I struggled along the road to recovery.

She was my inspiration, and the moment when I knew I had more respect and admiration for her than anyone else I'd ever met was when she asked the dietician to increase her meal plan so that she could gain weight quicker. She admitted that she was scared. She admitted that the voice was loud: it was screaming at her, it was protesting with a vengeance. But somehow she went against everything her mind was telling her to do, and she took a massive leap towards recovery. I looked up to Sammy like a big sister. I looked up to her as a hero, someone who I aspired to be.

After a few months as an inpatient Sammy was in a really good place. While I was still struggling immensely with the diet and gaining weight, she was handling it like a champion. She still found it undeniably hard, and she still had days where she believed that recovery was simply impossible, but the progress that she had made was incredible. So exceptional in fact, that she had reached a stage where she felt ready to go home. This is what I mean when I say she owned her recovery – she knew that the time had come when she could make a go of it on her own. She knew that the unit wasn't the best place for her anymore, and she fought for what she believed was the right way forward.

The time came for her to leave and in true Sammy style, she tried to sneak off first thing in the morning, before anyone else was up. She never wanted to make a fuss about anything – when she had her 30th birthday on the unit she refused to celebrate at all. She often kept her little victories to herself as much as possible so that no one made a big deal of them. But she couldn't escape me – I caught her trying to sneak off and I said to her what I said to everyone else as they got discharged: 'I'm so pleased for you that you get to go, but I wish you could stay here with me.' And I meant it – I was so happy that she got to go home to her loving husband and adorable dog, everything that she wanted, but I wasn't sure how I was going to keep going without her. She was my rock and now I had to brave the storm by myself. It was selfish, but I wanted her to stay so that she could continue to comfort me when I cried, tell me that everything was going to be okay when I believed the opposite.

We promised that we would stay in touch, message each other for support and comfort, and we did. We were still there for each other, even when we were miles apart. When she started to find things hard again at home I would stay up late at night so that she had someone to talk to. When the voices in her head once again became too loud to bear, I tried to drown them out by providing a voice of reason and warmth. We didn't talk every day, but we didn't need to: we knew that the other was there whenever we found ourselves needing reassurance or support.

As time went on I got the feeling that Sammy was struggling. She continued to give me all of the love and kindness that she had, but I knew that I couldn't give her the help that she really needed. I knew that she was having appointments with her medical professionals, and I knew that they were doing everything that they could to aid her recovery, but I still felt like I should have been able to do more. I told her that I was always there for her, I told her that she could message me any time she wanted, but I had limits. I couldn't see her in person, I couldn't give her therapy, and I wasn't a specialist in mental health. I hope she knew towards the end that if I could have cured her I wouldn't have hesitated for a second. I hope she knew that she was such a big inspiration not just to me, but to everyone on the unit – patients and staff alike. I hope she knew that she had made the hardest thing that I had ever gone through in my life just that little bit easier.

Sammy was a fighter. She was one of the strongest people I have ever known, and she never gave up, she didn't lose a single drop of her determination. In the end the eating disorder was just that little bit stronger. She had nothing to be ashamed of, and she had every reason to be proud of herself for all that she accomplished. When she was battling through the darkest time of her life, she gifted me light. When she was fighting through her own storm, she sheltered me from the rain. When she couldn't see a way forward, or she was unsure of which path to take, she guided me towards my freedom and away from any harm. Sammy didn't deserve to die. Sammy deserved to live her life to the fullest and enjoy every moment on offer. She never deserved to suffer for a single second or feel even a pin-prick of pain. Now that she's gone, I want to honour her memory by doing what I know she would have wanted from me – I want to destroy anorexia so that it can never hurt anyone again. I want to kick it and scream at it just how evil and despicable it is. I want to make the eating disorder suffer, I want to do everything that I can to hurt it, just like it hurts us.

I tell myself that Sammy's at peace now. She's no longer suffering, she's no longer feeling the cruel anguish that anorexia unleashes on its victims. I think it's true when people say that God chooses the best people, and he's been lucky enough to gain a true angel in Sammy.

Sammy, I hope you know just how incredible you are, I hope you know how loved you are, and I hope you know that you are my hero.

DEATH

Statistically, anorexia nervosa is the deadliest psychiatric disorder. Whether it be from the effects of malnutrition or from suicide, people suffering from anorexia are more likely to pass away than someone with any other mental illness. That's scary. I look back on the time when I was so poorly I couldn't move without my body protesting with aches and pains, and I'm in disbelief at how close to death I brought myself. I read in the newspapers that another beautiful soul has died from this godawful illness, and reading their story, I find stark similarities to my own experiences. It's humbling and it's shocking – the fact that I'm still here out of pure luck. I'm no stronger than anyone else, I'm much less brave than some of those who aren't with us anymore, yet for some reason my story continues while theirs is brought to a close. At one point I was told that a simple viral infection like the common cold, that my friends would be able to get over after a couple of days in bed, would probably end my life. I was told that if I fainted, I needed to ring an ambulance immediately. I was told when I was an inpatient that the reason why I couldn't use the stairs was because there was a chance of me having a heart attack if I did. The doctors didn't hold back on telling me what I needed to hear – I was told outright the risks of my illness, yet for a while I still chose not to eat, I still chose to face these dangers everyday and walk the tightrope between life and death.

I believed I was invincible, I believed that nothing could touch me. The chest pain I got when I'd been secretly exercising was nothing to worry about, the fact that I was hospitalised and fed through an NG tube didn't mean anything – I was so sure I wasn't going to die; that happened to other people, not me. I wasn't just being arrogant, I didn't think I was superior to other people, I just never believed that it would happen to me.

Anorexia knows I don't want to die, it knows I want to live my life to the fullest and make the most of what I have been gifted. So it tells me to just lose a little more weight, become a little more poorly, eat a little less and I'll be absolutely fine. It reassures me that nothing bad will happen, it tells me that I'm safe, but this is its way of keeping me trapped, its way of turning me against everyone who is trying to help me.

People do die from eating disorders. And those who manage to survive can be left with serious long-term health consequences. That's why it's so important that every time I'm not hungry, or I feel like skipping a meal, I have to remember that whatever the illness says about it being fine and however it manages to assure me that I won't be in danger, it is one hundred percent wrong. I have to remember Sammy, and all of the other courageous warriors that were taken from us too soon, and I have to listen to them cheering me on from that special place in Heaven where the most kind, caring, and loving people get to go. Even though their battles are over the war still rages on, and those of us left fighting are going to make them so proud. We're never going to let anorexia win, we're never going to give in to its outrageous demands or silly games. We will be strong, and we will fight with everything we have. I promise you, anorexia will not succeed.

PERIODS

Since I began restricting my food intake all of those months ago, my periods stopped. My body simply didn't have enough energy to reproduce anymore. It didn't have enough fat to make the hormones that it needed for a period to occur. I can't pretend that I wasn't pleased when I started missing periods, in fact the absence of them ended up being a motivating factor for me to continue to lose weight, to continue to hang on to the eating disorder. I always knew that recovery would bring my periods back, and it was the one aspect of recovery that I saw as a negative. I see people in recovery celebrating getting their periods back. Many of them are pleased that they have regained their fertility, many of them are pleased to have reached this huge recovery milestone. But for me that milestone was filled with fear and discomfort about my new body. My new, functioning body which was doing what it was supposed to do. My new body which no longer looked like a child, because it had once again become a woman.

The week that I realised my hormones were starting to come back, I found out what was happening by putting on a lot of weight; the very thing that I still feared the most. So I did what came naturally, and I burst into tears. I sobbed and wailed that I shouldn't have put that much weight on with what I'd eaten during the week. I was inconsolable. I was angry at my body, I was angry at my eating disorder, I was angry at all of the staff on the unit that told me to trust them because they knew what was right for me. But I had no reason to be angry - my body was finally healing, it was finally beginning to become whole again.

The hormones associated with periods cause the body to store extra water, and storing extra water will make that dreaded number on the scale go up. They also cause bloating, which proved to be an immensely scary aspect of recovery for me. Everybody told me that this 'weight gain' was temporary, that it would even itself out in the coming weeks, but it didn't make me feel any better. I was still terrified. I was convinced that they were wrong.

I was told a lot of times that my weight gain was

likely to be water retention; not one time did I truly believe it. I can't count the number of times that I was told that my weight gain was down to natural fluctuations, yet I still felt awful about myself and disgusted with my body. The scientific side of my mind knew it was true, I knew that weight was likely to have natural changes – water, hormones, even just the amount of urine in the bladder could cause weight to change. But it wasn't an acceptable excuse for anorexia – it was still determined to be angry with me.

Just as expected, a few weeks after my unsettling weight gain, my period returned. I'd tried not to think about it, I'd tried to put it out of my mind, but now it had become a reality. I was shaking and I was scared. My emotions threatened to overwhelm me, but I just about managed to keep it together. I felt like I should have been happy, I should have felt proud of myself for making so much progress, but by hitting this enormous breakthrough on my journey to recovery, I'd unlocked a whole new host of challenges to overcome.

The eating disorder convinced me that this was a definite sign that I was better. This meant that I didn't have to put on any more weight, I didn't have to eat as much anymore, I didn't have anorexia anymore. I felt healthy; for the first time in over a year, I felt normal. However I was still so stuck in this world of illness and suffering, that I didn't want to be normal. Being normal felt wrong and unnatural. I got strong urges to restrict – stronger than I'd had in months, and I told myself I was allowed to listen to them because I'd gotten my period back – I was practically recovered.

But even through the screaming of anorexia, I managed to fight the urges. I carried on just as I was doing, because deep down inside, I knew that I wasn't recovered. I was still underweight, and the fact that the thought of restricting my food intake even entered my head said that I still had an awful lot of work to do. This was yet another mountain to climb, another hurdle to overcome, but I knew that I would do it with the utmost bravery and determination, just like all of the other challenges I'd faced before.

'She sat back and allowed the world to turn. She let the fear, the terror, and the anxiety run through her, become one with her body and mind. And then she let it go. Then she became free.'

DISCHARGE

As I began to recover and gain weight I found it harder to see new patients come onto the unit. I saw their emaciated bodies and I missed my ropey muscles and my weak limbs. I grieved for my sick and skeletal self, I grieved for the aches all over my body and the pain I used to go through every single day.

I remember I was asked how I felt about my body, and I replied honestly, that I thought my body was the biggest on the unit. The look of shock that followed from the person who asked me stopped me in my tracks. She couldn't believe that I saw myself that way. She couldn't believe that the way in which I saw my body was so inaccurate, so different to reality. But there was no doubt in my mind over how I saw myself in the mirror, how I looked to other people. My calves were bigger than everyone else's on the unit, my chest was bigger than everyone else's. When I hugged other patients I could feel all of their bones sticking into me, but I knew that they weren't feeling the same from my body. Every time a new patient was admitted I had to fight through the voices, I had to overcome what almost felt like jealousy over their body. But I knew that I was on my own path to recovery. I knew that I had to follow my own road, because that was the only way I would ever survive.

As I became ever closer to being discharged, the tiny rebellious acts I took against Anorexia every day became the most important things in the world. Accidentally pouring 50ml too much milk for my breakfast and not pouring it back, or taking an extra spoonful of broccoli at tea. Choosing a bigger apple at lunch time because that was the one that looked nicer, despite the fact it would contain more calories. Each time I took a small step, whether it was just one potato or just one piece of pasta, I made huge leaps in my mind. Each victory was a solid reassurance that the real me was still in there somewhere, she was just waiting to be welcomed home. But before I could be discharged, I had to make a final push. I had to persevere through the last few challenges that would be thrown at me, and I would have to work more diligently than ever before.

The commitment and dedication I put in to those final few weeks repaid me in pure anxiety and unease. I was coming face to face with some of my biggest fears and conquering goals that I'd been holding on to for so long. I went to a café for snack and ate a luxurious salted caramel brownie, which was the most amazing thing I think I'd ever eaten. I bought a sandwich for lunch and got a huge packet of crisps with it which I devoured in minutes. I drenched my crumpets in butter so it dripped through the holes in the bottom, and I savoured every oily bite. Despite the unease and nervousness that came from these challenges, I was building skills ready to be free of the unit for good, to go home and continue everything that I'd worked so hard to achieve.

I was constantly getting closer to a healthy weight, and I could feel my body changing day by day. My legs were starting to get some shape around the thighs and calves, instead of being skinny, pale twigs. My shoulders were starting to broaden and my collar bones were no longer sticking out of my chest. I had a big, bloated recovery tummy which I resented, but which was a sign that I was doing the right thing. My life was finally getting back on track and I knew that I would be more than ready to return to university in nine months' time.

I still had progress to make, and I knew that I would still face enormous challenges while I was at home, but I also knew that I was ready. I was ready to become someone more than just the person with anorexia, or the girl with the eating disorder. I was ready to become Jade again.

Putting everything in place for my discharge date made it seem real, it made me acknowledge that this was really happening, and most of all it made me eager to prove that I could do this. Home leave had been starting to improve since that first difficult week, and I'd had much more practice at blocking anorexia out when it was shouting at me. Although I was still scared every time I gained weight, and I still felt my heart beating out of my chest every time I stepped on the scales, I'd started to become more relaxed around food. I'd even started to enjoy a few of my meals, which had once upon a time seemed like an impossibility. I was ready for discharge – I'd outgrown the inpatient unit and I was ready to spread my wings and fly for myself. I was ready to release my inner phoenix, rise from the ashes, and be born again.

Like every end, and every new beginning, there were always going to be things that I wished I could take with me into my new start. I wished that I could remain friends with the other patients for the rest of my life, because they were honestly some of the most supportive and understanding people I'd ever met. I wished that I could watch them grow and win against their own eating disorders, and I wished that I could see a day in the future where we would all meet up for a huge barbeque and eating disorders would be barred from entering the vicinity. But life doesn't work like that. Some relationships that mean the most to us can only be temporary, and I had to accept that although these people, patients and staff, had saved my life, they had to remain in the past and let me move on to make my own future.

The evening before I left the inpatient unit for the final time I felt utterly terrified. I was scared to leave everyone behind. I was scared to take control of my own recovery and become responsible for my own choices. I was scared to lose the eating disorder – something which however much I hated it, had become a huge part of me.

Although there were things I knew I would sorely miss about the inpatient unit, I also knew that there were many aspects that I wouldn't miss. I knew that by getting discharged I was gaining more than I'd ever had as an inpatient, like full independence, like strong family bonds, like the chance to have a lie-in and not have to be ready for medications by 8am (even on the weekend), like being able to go to the bathroom freely without it being locked most of the time. Not only was I gaining a life, I was gaining a job – I would only have a week to relax before I started work at a local café and bakery – and I was at last gaining hope and ambition. My goals from when I was first diagnosed – cake on my birthday and family dinner at Christmas, were back in the running, and I felt like I could do anything. I felt indestructible.

When I left the unit I was eating all of my meals and all of my snacks. I was gaining weight, and I was at a stage where I was deemed healthy enough and strong enough to go home to my family. But this was where the hard work really began, this is where I was left in the house by myself and I would have to face anorexia alone, with no one there to remind me of all of the reasons why I was fighting. I would have to choose what to eat every single day, and every single day I would have to choose recovery over the eating disorder, even though every fibre of my being was heading towards the eating disorder. I would have to be stronger than I'd ever been, and more resilient than I ever thought I could be.

My time at home began well - I would go to work after my breakfast and I would last until lunchtime without getting hungry or fatigued. I would be on my feet for hours every day, and although they ached when I got home, it was the good ache after a day of hard-work, not the awful ache after starving myself for months. I would eat my lunch every day without fail and whenever I felt the slightest urge to throw it away because I knew I could get away with it, I told the voice in my head to shut up and stop bothering me – this was my new life and I was going to do what made me healthy and happy.

Despite my optimism that being back at home would be the start of a perfect new chapter in my life, I eventually came to realise that anorexia was still hanging on to me everywhere I went. I was more able to avoid listening to the voice, but nothing could stop me from hearing it. I heard it telling me to eat less porridge, but I ignored it. I heard it telling me to put less cheese in my sandwich, yet I was able to defy it. But when it came to challenging my true fears, when it came to putting myself through that indescribable pain and distress in order to continue the fight, I really struggled.

Looking back there were so many signs that the eating disorder was still alive – when I refused to eat carbohydrates with my evening meal, when I became obsessed with how much exercise I was doing at work, the panic that I felt when someone offered me a tiny chocolate, the ridiculously scary thought of eating a sandwich from the café instead of my own packed lunch. Anorexia was still with me every minute of every day. Although I was winning, it was still fighting.

I was forever being told as an inpatient that people really struggle to put on weight when they go home, I was constantly being told that just maintaining my weight would be an excellent achievement. So when it came time to go home I felt so much pressure not to gain any more weight. I once again thought that if I gained weight I would be labelled as a someone who wasn't really ill. I would be pushed to the side, written off as someone who was doing fine, when in reality the voice was still with me every minute of every day.

Despite being on my feet for hours every day, despite eating less than I was on the unit, I still gained weight in the first few weeks after I was discharged. I felt like my body was failing me. My body was showing progress in recovery but my mind still felt trapped. There was a disconnect between what was going on in my head and what my weight was showing, however this disconnect was my body saving my life. This disconnect was my body doing what it needed to fully recover, in spite of everything I'd put it through, and everything I was still putting it through.

My body was never going to be happy until it was at its ideal weight, and that was still so far away. I *needed* to gain weight after I was discharged, I *needed* to continue the progress I'd made as an inpatient. Even though many people struggled after discharge, hadn't I proved that I wasn't 'many people?' Even if it would have been a huge achievement to just maintain my weight, this was my story, my journey. I had to do what was right for me, and that meant continuing to put on weight, even if it was a rarity. I had to stand up and fight for myself, advocate for myself. If that meant breaking the 'rules' and being outrageous, then so be it. I was ready to rebel.

ANOREXIA IN THE TIME OF COVID

One thing that I've neglected to mention so far in my story is the Covid pandemic and the impact that it had on my journey. I suppose that being shut off from the outside world made it all feel less real for me. The restrictions that completely changed everyone else's lives didn't have that much impact on me - I was already in hospital, I was already restricted to staying on the unit the majority of the time, I guess I was already in my very own 'lockdown' situation.

The one thing that did change for me was visitors. Every Sunday I would look forward to a visit from my family – we would chat, play board games, and just enjoy spending time in each other's company, but after a couple of months visitors were banned. The one good thing that I had to get me through every tough day, the one thing that was keeping me going when times got rough was taken away from me. Car trips off the ward ceased to happen, all of the reasons that I had to recover became no more. Home leave was no longer an option for anyone, regardless of where they were in treatment, and many of the exciting freedoms that came with getting off chair rest ground to a halt. I no longer had a reason to eat – the world had come to a standstill, and anorexia was the only thing that felt familiar, that felt somewhat safe in the chaos that was erupting all around us.

Although for me day to day living was relatively unchanged when the restrictions came into effect, I felt a definite shift in the atmosphere on the unit. Anxiety was prevalent, from worrying about people bringing the virus in, to worrying about food shortages and changes to the support we were receiving. In an already anxious population the distress was amplified by a thousand, and we all rebounded off each other's emotions. If one person was having a bad day, the mood would spread like wildfire through the patients and suddenly everyone was hopeless and miserable. But on the other hand, on good days we were unbeatable. We stood side by side supporting each other through thick and thin. A victory for one was a victory for all. We were one big machine, fighting anorexia together when hardship and suffering were plaguing the world.

Despite it being a truly horrific time for pretty much every person on the planet, throughout the pandemic I was grateful for so many things: I was grateful that I had a bed in an inpatient unit, and I was getting the best support through what was an awful time for many people both with and without mental illnesses; I was grateful that I was surrounded by people in a time when loneliness became a global crisis of its own; I was grateful that everyone who came in and out of the unit took precautions to protect us all from the awful illness which was ruining so many peoples' lives; I was grateful that the staff would show up to work everyday to look after us and make us smile, even in the darkest of times; I was grateful that even though I couldn't see my family in person, I was still able to speak to them everyday and I was grateful that they were safe; I was grateful that I was able to continue fighting my eating disorder, when so many people were unable to get the help that they deserved in an extremely challenging time.

I know without a doubt that my time in the unit would have been over quicker if it wasn't for the pandemic, but I also know that there's no point dwelling on something I can no longer change. What's important is that no matter how long and messy my journey ended up being, it still led to the same destination – recovery. In fact by taking a slightly longer route I learned more than I ever thought I would. I learnt the importance of patience and resilience. I learned that every time I had a bad day, I could get up the following morning and try again. I learnt that it was okay to fail, because failure meant that I was growing, and I was discovering more about myself and my strengths every day.

For months the whole country was made to stay home. Human contact became something of a distant memory and socialising became a thing of the past. The only stories on the news were of how many deaths there had been, and all of the interviews on breakfast television were asking people to speculate what would happen next on this long road through lockdown. Nothing felt real; I was convinced I'd wake up any minute and it would all have been a bad dream. Schools were closing, masks became mandatory, and travelling to a different county became illegal. It felt to me like the universe was breaking. It felt like I didn't know which way was up anymore, and I was trapped in this crazy world that no longer made any sense. Not only was I fighting against anorexia, I was doing it in a time when normal life was impossible. I was standing fearlessly and valiantly in the face of a demon when it was all that I could do to keep getting up in the morning.

But eventually, after a long and stressful period of uncertainty, unprecedented measures and widespread distress, things finally began to look up. Restrictions were easing and for me that meant I was allowed visitors again. I was limited to two visitors for up to one hour, sat outdoors and social distancing, all while wearing masks, and although it wasn't the ideal situation to find myself in, I was more than ecstatic just to see my parents in the flesh. Every week they would come without fail, making the three hour round trip just to see me for a short while, just to be with me and show their support. I was more thankful than I could ever express.

As the world slowly began its ascent out of the depths of despair, I followed it. I found my motivation to recover again, I was able to imagine a normal future for myself without the burden of anorexia, and I was able to dream once more. As the dark clouds which had enveloped the planet started to lift, I could see my way forward more clearly. I could see the stars guiding me home, and I could see the sun shining down just for me, telling me to keep holding on no matter how much I wanted to let go.

Because of the mayhem that Covid had inflicted upon the whole population, mental illness became a pandemic in itself. People were being made redundant, people who were living by themselves were getting lonelier by the day, and people who worked on the front line were putting themselves at risk every day to help everyone else get through this harrowing and nightmarish time. People who were recovering from eating disorders were relapsing, and people who had never experienced mental health issues in their lives were seeing a huge decline in the way that their mind coped with all of the hardship. The NHS was already completely overwhelmed, GP surgeries were struggling to deal with bigger pressures than they'd seen in years, and demand for mental health services was wildly increasing on an exponential scale.

At that time I was exceptionally lucky to be receiving help and support from my amazing mental health team, and I was truly blessed to be surrounded by people on the inpatient unit who never ever let what was going on in the world affect the way they cared for me. Somehow I managed to get through the first wave of the pandemic and the most intense part of my eating disorder and come out relatively unscathed, but it wasn't just my effort that allowed it to happen. The dedication of the people around me, all of the NHS workers, and every single stranger who gave me a smile on a bad day, or who spoke to me with kindness even though they couldn't see my battle, they made everything okay. They made me believe that the world could be compassionate and benevolent when it seemed to be throwing all of its misery my way. They made me believe in the greatness of humanity and the well-meaning nature of humankind. Most importantly, they made me believe in asking for help, because asking for help is strength. Seeking support at your worst will only show your resilience, and accepting assistance will only make you stronger.

MY 20 REASONS TO RECOVER

In the depths of an eating disorder, it can feel impossible to find motivation to recover. Everybody has different reasons, and it took me a long time to work out mine, but here are just a few of them:

- To get back to living my wonderful life
- To have energy to make memories and enjoy myself
- To not be cold, even in the winter
- To get my concentration back so I can smash my medical school exams
- To be able to walk up a flight of stairs without my legs feeling like they're going to drop off
- To have enough focus to read books and be able to escape into a million different

worlds
- To be able to run through the park after my beautiful dog
- To laugh, despite the voice telling me I'd never laugh again
- To be able to eat whatever I want, whenever I want and not have to feel guilty about something essential to life
- To have a healthy body that allows me to follow my dreams
- To be able to rest at the end of the day and get a good night's sleep, so I wake up refreshed and raring to go
- To go to the cinema and firstly, be able to concentrate throughout the whole film, and secondly, eat a whole sharing bag of chocolate to myself
- To go on a shopping spree and buy tons of new clothes that actually fit
- To bake some awesome cakes and tell people they can't have one because they're all mine
- To drive my car and have new adventures
- To join in with family meals and go out with friends, to feel like I truly belong
- To wear a bikini on the beach and not give a damn about my body
- To go on holiday and eat fish and chips dripping in salt and vinegar around the harbour

-     To go out to restaurants and choose whatever I want off the menu
-     To say, when people ask me what I'm most proud of in my life so far, that I kicked Anorexia's butt

DOWNHILL

Two weeks after my discharge from the unit I was a different person to who I was as an inpatient. I had a job which I loved and looked forward to every day, I smiled and I laughed and I made stupid jokes all the time, and I was happy. I still saw my psychologist every week but in between the appointments I wasn't thinking about anorexia, I was getting to know myself again. I was beginning to welcome back the girl who had lost her way, but who had fought tooth and nail to regain her life. I was beginning to recognise who I was without the eating disorder – the happy waitress who loved chatting to customers, and the aspiring doctor who was preparing to return to medical school.

Although things still weren't perfect – I was still struggling with a lot of foods and I was still obsessed with how much physical activity I was doing; I was beginning to recognise the real me taking pride of place in my mind. I was owning my recovery and I was showing the universe that I no longer needed an eating disorder to be happy in life.

For three weeks I managed to stay strong. For three weeks I was winning in the littlest of ways, and I felt like I was starting to triumph over the illness when it attempted to hold me back. I wasn't just 'the girl with the eating disorder' anymore, I was starting to really live my life the way I wanted to. Every day I was building up my strength and determination to get rid of anorexia for good.

But after mountains of hard work and resilience, came defeat. After all that suffering and heartache, came even more torture. Every ounce of hope and positivity that I was holding on to came crashing down around me and everything that I'd worked so hard for disappeared in a flash. I once again became trapped inside my mind with no way of escape.

It began on a Saturday. Rumours were spreading at work that the government were considering a second national lockdown due to Covid, and conversations were buzzing with anticipation about what would happen to all of our jobs. For everyone around me the nightmare that they'd already had to live through once was threatening to repeat itself, but for me this was unchartered territory. I was only just starting to get used to my new life and now it was being put in jeopardy, now I stood to lose it all. As soon as it was confirmed later that evening that there would be another lockdown, I began to panic – what would happen to my job? And more importantly (according to anorexia) – what was going to happen to my weight if I wasn't on my feet all day running around a café?

I was so caught up in worrying about the new restrictions that I never noticed the eating disorder creeping back up on me. I never noticed it worming its way surreptitiously back into my mind. So a couple of days later when I had an appointment with my psychologist and she weighed me, the fact that I'd gained even more weight than what I'd been gaining over the last few weeks was the final straw. If my weight was still increasing while I was doing so much physical activity, it was sure to rocket up as soon as I stopped going to work. I had to do something to halt it.

I drove home in a complete daze, disordered thoughts flooding my mind. Anorexia was convincing me that I had to restrict. It was calling me greedy, and selfish, and all the barbaric names under the sun and no matter what I did I couldn't drown it out. It taunted me for the rest of the day, reminding me of my weight gain with every mouthful of my tea. It made me irritable, it made me angry, and it made me sick with anxiety. It told me that tomorrow had to be different, tomorrow had to be 'better'. It told me that as long as I listened to it this time, everything would be okay. As long as I never betrayed it again, everything would work out.

I woke up the following morning on a mission to prove my loyalty to anorexia. From that day on the illness had control of me all over again. From that day on it ruled my life just like it had done before. It was like a switch was flicked inside my brain and one day I was eating everything on my meal plan, the next day the fear came flooding back and my only thoughts centred on my weight and my eating. The last couple of days at work before everything was stopped, I was completely preoccupied with the war raging in my head. I knew I had all of these brilliant qualities – I was kind, I was smart, and I was caring, so why was starving my body the only way I could appreciate myself? Why was punishing and torturing myself the only way that I could vaguely like who I was? It made no sense, yet to me it felt like my future was clear – the eating disorder was right all along, I couldn't live without it, I was weak and I was pathetic and without it I was nothing. In the space of a day I had reverted right back to those damaging behaviours which were only bound to lead in one direction - down.

Over the next few weeks my mood went down, my weight went down, and my prospects went down. Coming out of the second lockdown after four long weeks, I hoped and prayed that the café where I worked remained closed, because I had gotten myself into such a state that there was no way I could go back to work. I knew that I was yet again putting my return to university in jeopardy, but I didn't care. I could only think about the next day, or at most the next week; the future meant nothing to me anymore.

I went right back to where I'd started – cold, hungry, weak, and miserable, and that was just me. It destroyed my parents to see me go through the same hell again when I'd put in so much effort to escape the first time, and it devastated them to know that there was nothing they could do to help me. Anorexia kept telling me to just lose one more kilo and that would be it, then it'd be happy. But it was never happy. Eating disorders will only feel happy when you are on your death bed and it's too late to stop the inevitable. Eating disorders will only be happy when they know that there's no way that you can beat them, and the only way to make sure of that is to kill the opposition. I went from eating cheese sandwiches every day for lunch, to becoming terrified if I cut slightly more cucumber than normal. I went from eating a big bowl of porridge and two slices of toast for breakfast every day, to worrying about whether an extra carrot stick would make me gain weight.

Anorexia once again became all-consuming. It erased all logical thought in my brain and replaced it with fear and distress. It didn't allow room for anything else, it became my life and it became me.

As time went on my two ultimate aims – birthday cake and Christmas dinner, came and went yet again with no hint of accomplishment. Once again these special days were ruined by my illness and there was nothing I could do to escape for just a few hours. It categorically refused to leave me alone to let me celebrate and have a good time with my family, and it hung over us like a dark cloud that refused to budge. How I wish I could have blown that dark cloud away to reveal the blue skies hiding behind it. But if eating disorders were that easy to conquer there would be no need to feed people through tubes, and there would be nobody losing their lives due to anorexia's reign of terror. The world would be a much happier and brighter place.

Every time I went to see my psychologist or psychiatrist and they told me I needed to eat more I nodded in agreement. I told them that I would make changes, but in my head I knew that I wasn't telling the truth. There was no way I was going to do what they were suggesting – anorexia wasn't ready to be banished from my mind again and I wasn't ready to lose it. I became a master of telling people what they wanted to hear. I became a master of deceiving everyone around me, and while I felt incredibly guilty, the eating disorder was congratulating me on managing to lie to anyone who was trying to help me.

When talk of going back to the inpatient unit began to surface I never believed it would become a reality. I never believed I would end up back where I had worked so hard to escape from. I had so many reasons to avoid another admission, so many reasons why I never wanted to go back – the lack of independence, the lack of control over my diet, the lack of freedom, but none of those reasons were enough to make me start eating properly again. I tried, I really tried. I tried to increase my porridge by five grams, just five extra grams of oats, but the anxiety was too much. I tried to have more salad with my tea, but anorexia berated me for being greedy and never went quiet. I tried to turn it around, but I was exhausted. I was simply too tired to fight anymore.

So when I was offered a bed on the same inpatient unit only three months after I'd left, I caved. The illness wanted me to stay strong, it wanted me to stay a thousand miles away from the place where it knew it would be defeated, but I couldn't go on by myself any longer. I'd been through all this before and I knew that the only way forward would be to seek the support of the inpatient unit, I knew that I had to relinquish the control I was so desperately trying to hang on to. So feeling considerably too well to be admitted, and knowing that I was signing up for another brutal, gruelling ride, I took one of the bravest steps I ever took. I once again accepted help.

Dear Jade,

I know you're hurting, but I promise that the pain will pass. I know you feel like letting go, but I promise that everything will be worth it in the end. I know you feel beaten and broken down by life, but I promise you that it will get better.

Right now I know you're struggling to see a future in which you're free of the eating disorder. I know that you imagine eating normally, and the thought is so terrifying, so overwhelming that you immediately try to picture something else, anything else to take your mind off the battles you have yet to face. But it doesn't matter if you can't see that far into the future, as long as you can see your next step, that's enough.

You have no idea how courageous you really are. To go through what you've been through, to endure what you've had to endure and come out of the other side still fighting, is truly amazing. It may not always feel like it, but you can do anything you put your mind to. Never give up.

AUTISM

Throughout my life, I've always had my quirks – I've always struggled to make friends; I HATE going out in the evening and at night; if I go to a concert or watch a funny film my face will remain straight throughout, even if it's the funniest thing I've ever watched; I get extreme anxiety if I believe I'm going to be late for something; I absolutely love smelling things – shower gels, candles, food; and I am in love with socks, and have hundreds of pairs which I refuse to throw away. In short, I've always thought of myself as 'weird'. Throughout my life I've made an effort to suppress my 'quirks'. I've made an effort to conform to what society would view as 'normal'. But just before I was admitted to the inpatient unit again, a diagnosis of autism spectrum disorder not only explained these quirks, but it set me free.

As soon as I was given the screening

questionnaire by my psychiatrist, I knew that it was leading somewhere – as I read through the questions I felt like they were aimed directly at me. As I read them I found that they were putting the things that I thought were weird about me into words. With each question my life began to make more sense. And when I scored highly on the questionnaire and was asked to have an assessment, although I was worried and anxious about where it might lead, I also knew that it could make me fly.

Alongside my other quirks, I've also always been very particular about how I like my food. For as long as I can remember, I've never liked different food groups touching on my plate; I've always been very particular about textures of foods; I've always hated eating hot and cold foods together, like fries and ketchup; and I've always avoided eating what I perceived as 'wet' and 'dry' foods together. When I was younger I was always labelled as a fussy eater, and perhaps I was. But it's left me wondering whether these behaviours made me more predisposed to suffering with an eating disorder, whether these behaviours somehow influenced my later struggles.

There were too many times to count during my first inpatient admission when these behaviours were mistaken as features of the eating disorder. I would become increasingly frustrated with the staff as they tried to force me to eat differently to how I'd eaten my whole life. I knew that I'd been doing these things since I was a small child, and I knew that I found it impossible to eat differently, but I couldn't understand why. I couldn't understand why I was so intent on using these safety nets during my meals. That was until I got the diagnosis that changed my life.

When the psychologist said the words: 'you meet the criteria to be diagnosed with autism spectrum disorder', I felt nothing but relief. I knew that this wasn't going to change who I was, it was just going to make me more confident. It was going to make me more aware of my anxieties and make me more equipped to control them. My diagnosis gave me permission to go around the supermarket smelling all the shampoos before I chose one to buy. It gave me permission to turn up to places ridiculously early to prevent me panicking that I was going to be late. It gave me permission to eat my lunch off three different plates because I didn't want things mixing. It meant that I could get ten pairs of socks for my birthday because everyone knew that's what I loved. I finally had permission to be me.

Most importantly, I knew my diagnosis would lead to big changes in the way that I recovered from my eating disorder. It not only helped me to gain more understanding of how my illness first came about, it helped me to express my worries and concerns better. It helped other people to understand me and understand that I couldn't always put my feelings into words. It helped me to distinguish which of my behaviours around food were due to the eating disorder, and which were due to autism, and I got chance to work with mental health professionals who helped me to understand myself and live life to the full.

As time went on I became more in tune with my anxieties, and I learnt more about myself than ever before. Heading into my second admission I knew that it was going to be different from last time. I knew that this next admission would be better, because I was equipped with a better understanding of who I was. I was finally able to accept myself, now I just had to learn to love myself.

'And through the storm she stumbled, each step ten times harder than the last. Yet still she moved forwards, still she persevered, because she knew that the light was waiting for her on the other side.'

INPATIENT AGAIN

Travelling to the inpatient unit again, which was a trip I made so many times going to and from home leave, was almost too familiar. I didn't want to be someone who fought with eating disorders their whole life, I didn't want to spend my future going back and forth between units never quite making a full recovery, I wanted a life without this hanging over me. I wanted to live, properly and wholly, without anything holding me back.

I spent a lot of time contemplating over what went wrong the last time I attempted recovery. I spent a lot of time planning what I could do differently the second time around, and the answer was, I eventually realised, I had to do this for me. No more eating just to get discharged, I was recovering to give myself a better life. I was recovering for me. I knew that although I was in a much better place when I was last discharged, I was still counting calories, I was still restricting my intake, and I was still absolutely terrified of making my own choices around food. I realised that when I was in control of my own diet, weight gain came with a thousand times more guilt than when somebody else decided what I ate. I realised that I had to learn to accept the consequences of my actions and take responsibility for my choices.

Last time I was an inpatient I would watch new people come onto the unit and eat straight away. I would compare them to myself and see so much bravery and commitment, while all I saw in myself was weakness. It took me months before I began to eat everything on my plate, it took me months to begin to make any type of progress on this long and winding path. I swore that if I had the chance to go back and start recovery again I would just eat and eat and not care what anyone else thought, I wouldn't care if people thought I was greedy, I would simply do what I had to do to stop the pain and suffering careering through my mind.

So at the beginning of this second shot at beating anorexia, I made a promise to myself. I promised myself that I would eat whatever was put in front of me, because I knew that delaying the weight gain was simply wasting time and prolonging the inevitable. I promised myself that I would get discharged and back home as quickly as possible, so that I could prepare to go back to medical school. I promised myself that I would go through all of the pain, all of the heartache, and all of the torment because that was the only way to rid myself of the monster inside me.

The second time I knew I was going away I packed my suitcase as if I was going for a week on holiday. I took nothing to decorate my room, I took a minimal amount of clothes, I took hardly anything to keep me occupied; I was sure I'd be out before I knew it. I was sure it would be so different this time, I was sure I would just eat everything that was presented to me and be out before I knew it.

My first meal back on the unit was half a slice of toast with a spoonful of baked beans. I'm sure to all of the staff it looked like a pathetic lunch, but when it was presented to me my panicked mind instantly started comparing it to my lunch at home. How many more calories were in this? Was this alone going to make me gain weight? To me it wasn't pathetic – it was a massive mountain that I had to climb.

In the back of my mind the promises that I had made to myself were trying to grab my attention, but the anorexia was louder. It was telling me that I wasn't poorly enough to be admitted. It was telling me that there were so many other people that needed help more than me, and it was telling me that the only way to be worthy of help was to continue to lose weight. None of this was true. All of the staff were telling me that none of this was true, but I didn't believe them, the illness didn't believe them. It was just me and the eating disorder back together again, fighting against everyone who wanted me to get better.

When I looked at that tiny portion of beans on toast all I knew was that I wasn't allowed to eat it. I couldn't distinguish the voices in my head, I couldn't dissect who was saying what, I couldn't think clearly enough to rationalise what was going on, I only heard that if I ate the food on that plate something awful would happen. I could feel the adrenaline running through my veins, I could feel the threat of the food forcing my body into fight or flight mode. All the memories of my last admission came flooding back – the tears, the wobbles, the anxiety – I didn't know if I could do this all over again; it was just too damn hard.

I tried my best with my meal but after it was taken away I broke down and cried. I cried for myself, for having to fight this again, and I cried for everyone else who was suffering – I wish more than anything that mental illness didn't exist, I wish I never had reason to enter this cruel and vicious world. I wish that recovery could be as simple as taking a pill and getting better, but anorexia demands excruciating, back-breaking work from anyone wishing to beat it. It demands full-time commitment and nothing but ultimate dedication from those who take it on, and still it fights back with every ounce of hate that it has. Still it sets out to destroy its foe, and if it goes down, its victim goes down too.

The promises that I made to myself were a lot easier said than done. I thought myself weak for not being able to beat the eating disorder properly last time. I felt ashamed for having failed at something that had looked so promising. But my second admission taught me that where I thought I was weak, I was actually strong for making as much progress as I had against a horrific force. Where I was ashamed, I should have been proud for reaching out for help and being prepared to fight once more. Even though I promised that this time would be different, that this time would be better, the second time was every bit as hard as the first.

It's easy to look back and be hard on myself for giving up too easily, for not being resilient enough, for not holding on just that little bit longer when I felt like quitting. But nothing can quite describe with enough clarity just how draining, and just how impossible it feels to fight against yourself every minute of every day. Nothing can compare to having to rise each morning knowing that your own mind is going to put you through hell, but deciding to stand tall and face the day anyway. The trick is to know that while it all feels impossible, you are capable of amazing things, and one of those amazing things is to get through everything you thought to be too hard with grace and dignity, and you can prove yourself, and the eating disorder, and everyone who said you couldn't do it, completely wrong.

I knew that this time I would gain weight quicker. I knew that I wasn't going to mess around for months trying to remain dangerously underweight. I mentally prepared myself for what was going to happen – I told myself that I'd accept my fate, whatever it may be. But although I'd been through it plenty of times before, although it didn't come as a surprise when it happened, the second time I began to gain weight again destroyed me.

It wasn't the biggest gain I'd ever been through, but it was by far the most distressing. Before I stepped on the scales I was hesitant; I knew what was going to happen, I was just trying desperately to hang onto that last thread of hope that I was mistaken. The nurse sitting beside me looked into my eyes and he told me that whatever I was dreading, whatever I was thinking was going to happen, it wouldn't. And like a fool, I believed him, I let him convince me that I was about to be proven wrong. So I went and did everything that my mind was begging me not to do, and I let myself be weighed.

Immediately after I'd stepped down from the scale I felt the same as ever before – panicked, but with the knowledge that it would pass, with the knowledge that the pain would only be temporary. But then I became angry. Angry at myself, angry at my body, angry at the nurse. How dare he tell me that all my fears were unfounded? How dare he reassure me that everything would be fine when he had no idea? I was supposed to trust these people but they lied. They lied to me, telling me that I wouldn't put on lots of weight, but I proved them wrong. I knew my body better than anybody else and I vowed never to trust the doctors or the nurses or the dietician ever again. At least that's what I felt in the moment.

Over time the anger ebbed away and I found myself able to begin trusting again, but I still hold the belief that I know my body better than anyone. I still find myself doubting the professionals. It doesn't mean that I don't listen to what they say, it just means that I take ownership of my own recovery. It means that I advocate for what I know is best for me. But that day I was completely caught up in my eating disorder. That day I didn't see weetabix and toast for breakfast, I saw calories and weight gain and the most awful consequences. I didn't see jacket potato and cheese and beans for lunch, I saw fear and danger and panic enveloping me. I think I cried so much that day that I ran out of tears. By the time the burger and chips was presented at tea I had nothing left to give. No energy, no fight, no hope. When I was found in my room by one of the support workers an hour after I'd left the dining table in tears, sat calmly and quietly in my chair, bright red blood slowly dripping to the floor from the self-inflicted wounds to my arm, I felt nothing. I had no emotion left inside of me. I'd simply had enough, I simply wished that I didn't have to feel this pain anymore.

Dear Jade,

The only way to beat this thing is to listen to it screaming in your head, and then do the complete opposite of what it says. Because every time you let that voice take control, it is winning. It is wearing you down little by little.

Take every horrible thought as a challenge. If it's telling you that you can't do it, or you're not allowed, it's actually the most important thing you have to do. It won't be easy, and it will hurt, but that's how you know you are succeeding. And I promise you, the pain won't last.

You are allowed to curse at the world for putting you through this. You are allowed to let your mind and body rest. You are allowed to have a complete breakdown and want to give up. But you must get back on your feet and keep fighting. You are allowed to gain weight, you are allowed to eat ANYTHING you want, and you are allowed to be wholly, unapologetically you.

Please don't hurt yourself, you deserve to be free from pain, mentally and physically. Please don't be so hard on yourself, you are being brave just for getting up everyday and carrying on. Please keep fighting, because you are so worth it.

You have suffered enough in this war with yourself and you deserve to win. Just hold on for a little longer

JADE KIDGER

– you can do it, you brave little fighter.

HAPPY PLACE

During each and every meal that I fight through, I become detached from reality, and I imagine my happy place – on the beach with my family.

We've taken a delicious picnic in the cool-bag and as the midday sun blazes overhead, we decide it's time to eat. My Mum pulls out lovingly-made sandwiches which were prepared that morning, with fruit, crisps, and little extra treats: sausage rolls, scotch eggs, mini pork pies. It's a feast, and everyone eats until their hearts are content. I savour each and every mouthful as I try not to contaminate my food with sand. The smell of suncream mixes with the aromas coming from the food and although they shouldn't go together, the smell reminds me of every holiday I've ever been on.

I'm looking forward to blissfully reading my book

for a couple more hours, until we get ice-creams as a mid-afternoon treat. I think I'll either go for salted caramel or chocolate – I haven't quite decided yet, but I know that it'll be delicious, and I won't have any regrets, any guilt, or any anxiety. Not even later when we eat fish and chips around the harbour for tea. Not even when my huge portion gets lashings of salt and vinegar, because that's how I like to eat my chips. Not even when we go back to the cottage we've rented and we tuck into more food – chocolate and sweets and crisps. Life is good. I am free.

But there's always something to pull me out of this trance that I get myself into. In the back of my head there's always the reminder that instead of being on the beach, I'm stuck in an inpatient unit trying to fight my way through a bacon sandwich. My wild imagination takes my mind off reality for a few minutes, but it will always, without fail, come crashing back.

Nevertheless, imagining I'm on the beach with my family helps me to get through each meal. It helps me to remember who I am and why I'm doing this. It reminds me that a future is possible, a future without the eating disorder.

COPING MECHANISMS

After overcoming the initial hurdles that I faced at the start of my second admission, I ate. I ate pizza, I ate chocolate, I ate potatoes. Everyone told me I was doing so well but they couldn't hear what was going on inside my head. On the surface everything looked brilliant, but inside the eating disorder was louder than it had ever been before. It made it known that there'd be a punishment for eating, it made it known that it expected me to sacrifice another part of my soul to it in return for nourishment, and it wasn't long before it demanded penance.

The first time I punctured my skin and saw a bloom of red appear on my arm, I was relieved. When I felt that sharp sting I knew that I had served my sentence for that day. I had repaid any debts I had involving the eating disorder and I was absolved from my sins. So I did it again. And again, and again. Every time a new wound appeared on my skin I was marking the eating disorder in indelible ink. They could take away the weight loss, they could take away my bony hips and my protruding collar bones, but this was something that was mine, and mine alone. Nobody could remove this from me, nobody could deprive me of the suffering and the scars that I was inflicting upon myself.

For a while it was my dark little secret. I would roll my sleeves down over the damage that I had done and I would carry on like nothing had happened – I went to the dining room and ate my yoghurt, and all the while the stinging pain was reminding me that I was allowed to eat, because I'd paid anorexia in another way.

The secrecy thrilled me, the intimacy between anorexia and I grew and grew and our bond became stronger until we were one. Yes it hurt, but I deserved the pain; it was my punishment for giving in to temptation and eating. At least that was what it told me. As I drifted towards sleep in bed that first night, my throbbing arm wrapped in a towel to stop it bleeding over the bedsheets, I truly believed every word that anorexia was muttering to my vulnerable, exhausted mind. I believed that injuring myself was my sentence for daring to survive. I believed that I was required to make payment in order to carry out a basic human need. Worst of all, I believed the illness was my friend.

That first day, I'd never felt anything close to the relief that temporarily filled me when I felt the pain. I thought I'd cracked the secret to recovery. I thought I'd finally found a way through the hell of anorexia. But what happens the next day when the eating disorder demands that you cut yourself more but you don't want to? What happens when you try to fulfil the darkest wishes of your mind but this time the pain is torture, too intense to bear? You feel weak. You feel like a failure. You don't want to hurt yourself anymore but it doesn't matter what you think. You are merely a slave to anorexia now, it demands to hurt, so you must hurt. It demands suffering, so you must suffer.

I would drag my feet up the stairs to the privacy of my bedroom as slowly as I possibly could, trying to postpone the moment where I would feel compelled to abuse myself in the name of anorexia. I would make sure that I was ready to hide what I was doing should anyone enter my room, because despite pleasing the eating disorder, I felt 'naughty'. I felt like I was doing something wrong, despite the fact that my mind was telling me it was one hundred percent right. But I couldn't trust my mind; I couldn't trust myself any more.

I realised that I'd gotten myself into something terrible, I knew that I'd found my new downfall, but it was already too late. I'd gotten myself in too deep from the moment I'd listened to anorexia and unleashed this newfound violence and cruelty upon myself. It was just one more way of showing my body the hate I believed it deserved. It was just one more way of trying to redeem myself for sins that never even existed.

I couldn't stop, no matter how hard I tried. Any time that I was sat in the lounge relaxing, watching TV, or reading my book, the need to hurt myself overwhelmed me. Through the calmness of my surroundings anorexia would scream obscenities at me, demanding that I go and pay it what I owed, demanding that I showed it my unwavering commitment and loyalty. That loyalty included keeping my actions to myself, not allowing anyone in on our secret, not allowing anyone to save me from this hell I'd gotten myself into.

I struggled to make sense of what was going on in my head. I was constantly asked what was happening in my mind when the staff could see I was in distress, and every time I would get more and more frustrated because I couldn't put into words what I was feeling. Mostly I think I just felt empty. I knew there was pain and torture inside me but they were buried too deep to grab hold of.

Self-harming gave me a way of understanding myself. If I was in pain on the outside, I was no longer thinking about the pain on the inside. If I was in pain on the outside, it gave me a reason to be suffering and to take care of myself. I suppose it was my way of showing myself and the rest of the world what was going on in my head. The violence that I inflicted upon myself represented the anger and aggression that came from anorexia. The often-excruciating pain stopped me from feeling numb; it allowed me to translate my thoughts into actions which were so much easier to interpret. Every time a drop of blood left my body it represented my tears, tears which the eating disorder rarely let me show to other people. Every line represented the hurt which was consuming me. Every scar represented the battles that I'd faced, no matter whether I'd won or lost.

Despite self-harm serving a purpose for me, it wasn't pretty, it wasn't strong, and it wasn't a good way to deal with my feelings. It left me so sore that some days I could barely move. It left me terrified to have a shower because I dreaded getting warm water in the wounds. It left me waking up every morning feeling so ashamed that I'd yet again got blood on the bed sheets. It left me with infections so bad that I could hardly walk or stand up. It left me fed up, it left me exhausted, and it left me feeling like a monster.

I secretly prayed that someone would notice what I was doing to myself and help me stop. Of course, the right thing to do would have been to confide in someone, but anorexia forbade that. My secret was finally revealed when I went to get weighed in my nightie one morning. It was the first time I'd let anyone see my bare arms since I'd started unleashing all of my feelings onto my skin, and weirdly, the relief I felt that someone else was now in on my secret was almost akin to the relief that I felt when I first cut myself.

The eating disorder was cursing me for letting someone see, for threatening its reign of terror, but I could also hear praise somewhere inside me. Praise for being brave enough to ask for help, for being fearless enough to stand up to the eating disorder. I was more than willing to give up what I'd been using to do the damage, in fact I couldn't wait for someone to take it from me, to rid me of the means to harm myself. I thought that if I didn't have anything to use it would be easier, the urge would be weaker, but that turned out not to be true.

As soon as I handed over what I'd been using, my brain went into panic mode – it panicked that the marks would disappear and I'd be left with nothing, it panicked that I'd have no way to rid myself of my guilt and all of the other feelings swirling around my head. I felt compelled to go straight up to my bedroom and search through all of my belongings in order to find something else sharp to use. It didn't matter what it was, as long as it was sufficient to break my skin and produce the deep red marks I'd come to hold on to like a comfort blanket throughout my mess of a life.

So began the cycle of feeling rubbish, so turning to self-harm, then feeling even worse about myself when people noticed, so turning to self-harm even more. Even when I'd given up all the sharps in my possession I still managed to find something else to use, even when I swore I'd stop and I knew I'd had enough I couldn't break the vicious, never-ending cycle of self-destruction.

Anorexia told me that I was letting people see what I'd done on purpose. It convinced me that I was a selfish attention-seeker who wanted nothing more than to make people worry about her even more than they already were. I felt even more like a fraud, and I felt worse about myself than I ever thought I could feel. I hated what I had become. I hated my body, I hated my mind, and most of all I hated anorexia.

My life became so dark and so horrendous that no matter how hard I tried, I couldn't see a single spark of light. I would sit in bed throughout the night trying to formulate a plan in my mind of how to end it all, trying to determine which way would be best to escape from the dire reality that my life had become. I knew that I simply couldn't go on like I was – loyally serving the eating disorder everything that it asked of me, bearing my soul for the monster to chip away at until I was nothing. I was beaten. I had given up all optimism and all hope of recovery. The only thing I could do now was survive the days until I had enough courage to save myself from my misery, until I granted anorexia its ultimate wish of destroying me for good.

SELF-HARM

Self-harm isn't glamorous or attractive, self-harm is feeling so distressed that you believe the only way to survive is to cause yourself immeasurable pain and agony. Self-harm is screaming and sobbing while you try so hard not to surrender to the urges, and thinking yourself weak when you give in. Self-harm is feeling so broken by life, that you feel the only way to cope is to torture and maim yourself.

It soon becomes an addiction. You want to stop with every fibre of your being, but your mind is too strong. Your mind demands that you continue to cause yourself unspeakable pain. You feel powerless, you can no longer control your own body. You have danced with the devil, but he refuses to let you go.

I know that self-harm doesn't make me strong, I am strong despite my struggles. I know that it doesn't make me beautiful, I am beautiful despite my scars. Self-harm was my way of coping, but it is toxic. It has caused me more suffering than I ever could have imagined. It is dangerous and it is unforgiving.

Nobody on this planet should ever feel like they have to cause themself pain. Nobody should ever feel so distressed or so broken that they feel the only way forward is to cause themself terrible harm. It breaks my heart to know that other people go through this, it breaks my heart knowing that other people have to feel the same agony as I do. Having to constantly battle against your own mind is a torture that I wish never existed. A torture that I am determined to beat.

'And from all of the pain and all of the hurt, emerged a warrior. Yes, she was broken, and yes, she was imperfect, but nevertheless, she was beautiful.'

ANOTHER STORM, ANOTHER FIGHT

How could I be stupid enough to put myself through recovery all over again? How could I erase all of my hard work from my last admission in a matter of months and put myself back to the beginning of the toughest fight of my life? I never ever considered that recovery could be as hard as it is. I wildly underestimated the strength and the resilience that I would need in order to scrape back the remaining remnants of my life.

Every time I wanted to give up I had to dig deeper than ever before, and somehow find the courage to carry on living through the torment and anguish that was casting immovable and impenetrable shadows over my mind. Yet somehow I did it. Somehow, on the gloomiest of days and the darkest of nights, I agonisingly pulled myself towards the smallest glimmer of hope imaginable. Somehow I survived, when my eating disorder was trying it's damn hardest to kill me.

Each day that passed was an achievement. Each week that my plan to end my suffering failed to become a reality, I was dragged ever further away from the dangers of my own head. It was painstakingly slow, but I started to believe there was a way out of this war that had been going on for far too long. I was so tired. I was beaten and I was worn down, but still I saw a chance, however slim it was, to save myself once more. I fought with every fibre of my being; each mouthful was agony and each meal brought with it excruciating torture. I began to be able to withstand the urges to harm myself. I began to learn that I didn't owe anorexia anything – I was allowed to eat without punishing myself.

Slowly, ever so slowly, I tiptoed my way forwards out of the hell that had become my existence. I thought that the second time would be easier. I knew what to expect: the overwhelming feelings of guilt and greed when I managed to complete a meal, the sheer panic and self-loathing that came with weight gain, the mental and physical exhaustion that came hand in hand with fighting for your life every single day. But each war is so different. Each battle brings unique challenges, and nothing can prepare you for those unexpected hits that wound you so deeply.

I still cried when I gained weight. I still felt pure panic when I was presented with certain foods. I still curled up in my blanket and wished so hard that everything would just go away. The road was long and winding, the days terrifying and unpredictable, yet still I survived. Still I got up every day and smiled and cracked jokes at the table; still I talked about my future at university with pure passion, even though the hope of going back was fading away; still I pretended everything was okay, when inside I was barely holding on.

While I was on the unit, I would go to great lengths to hide my true feelings. When I cried I did it in my room, alone. When I'd had enough and I didn't think I could go on anymore I would force myself to laugh, to be the 'happy one', the 'strong one'. Anorexia wouldn't let me show weakness. It wouldn't let me be vulnerable, it wanted me to suffer alone, with no one to comfort me or tell me that everything would be okay. It wanted me all to itself, to bully and taunt until I believed that I was nothing. If I wasn't the sickest or the thinnest person I wasn't good enough. If my eating disorder wasn't the most serious, I hadn't been working hard enough.

The illness made me believe everything it told me, but I couldn't voice my thoughts to anyone – they were embarrassing, they were 'wrong', and they were completely irrational. I was surrounded by other patients, nurses, support workers, yet I was so lonely. I thought that nobody on Earth could have any clue how I was feeling. I thought that I alone was suffering these nonsensical ideas. But here's what I wish someone would have told me at the time: 'You are not alone. Yes, the anorexia is making you feel alone, but so many people are here for you, rooting for you, cheering you on from the sidelines. You may feel like you're by yourself on the frontline, fighting solo, but what you can't see is the army behind you. Defending you against the enemy, holding you up when you can barely stand, bringing you home to keep you safe, to keep you warm. You are not alone.'

SAVING A LIFE

Every single day that I got out of bed during recovery, I went downstairs to the dining room, and I saved my own life. I think it's a dream that everyone has – to be able to save someone's life. To catch someone as they fall, to bring someone back from the brink of death, to protect someone when blows are raining down on them. What I think most people don't realise is you don't need to perform these big acts of heroism to save someone; you can start with yourself.

Saving your own life is just as valid, just as important, and just as heroic as any one of those acts. Consistently winning the battle against a dark force that's only wish is to kill you is inspirational, it is extraordinary, it is incredible. It's a shame that society doesn't seem to acknowledge these achievements with the same declarations of outstanding bravery and immense fearlessness as other life-saving efforts.

But know this – I see you. I'm so very proud of everything that you're fighting against, and even though it's so hard, and even though you might not feel like you've achieved much, I know that every day you survive is a battle won. I know that every meal that you attempt is a defiance against the eating disorder. So carry on going. You can do this.

I SEE THE LIGHT

Once again, through the intense pressures of inpatient treatment, the looming threats of my future career aspirations being taken away from me, and my sheer resilience and strength, I made it through the crippling darkness and I once again began to see brighter days ahead.

I came to the realisation that I wanted to be rid of my eating disorder in the future more than anything. I wanted to go on holidays and eat ice cream on the beach and fish and chips on the seafront and sweets on the long journey back, just like the rest of my family. I wanted to stuff my face with so much chocolate and turkey and pigs in blankets at Christmas that I couldn't possibly eat another mouthful more. I wanted to be free to have cake on my birthday, to accept food from people when they offered and not feel guilty, to not worry all the time about what I was eating, what my weight was doing.

But despite knowing exactly what I wanted and exactly how to get there, something huge stood in my way - the word 'future' was holding me back. I wanted all of these things so much, but I wanted them in time. I wanted them at some point, but not at that exact moment. What I wanted in that exact moment was to cling on to my eating disorder with both hands and never let go. What I wanted in that moment was my thin, emaciated body back that I had when my weight was so low. What I wanted right then was to suffer, to suffer and agonise over every little thing I ate, every tiny bit of exercise I did until it drove me crazy.

There was never a time when I felt ready to recover. The eating disorder was forever telling me that I couldn't recover because I wasn't thin enough yet, my BMI was still too high, or I wasn't sick enough, wasn't hurt enough, wasn't weak enough. Every single excuse for not recovering came from my eating disorder. The wish for the return of my old body, the instinct to hang on to the thing that was torturing me for as long as possible, the anxiety that I so yearned to stay with me; these things were all implanted into my head by anorexia, yet I still believed that they were my thoughts, my feelings.

I came to understand that recovery was a

process. It was a long, rocky path that had ups, downs, successes, and many many frustrations. I learned that it would take time to heal, some days recovery would be eating doughnuts and cheesecake and making memories with my family, and other days recovery would be struggling to get out of bed, crying my way through the day and cursing the demon that brought me all this pain. It wasn't as easy as a simple flick of a switch like I once thought – one day I was ill and starving myself, the next day my illness was cured because I ate everything on my meal plan and more. In reality recovery is much more complex, much more confusing, and it has a million different appearances.

There was never a day when I believed that it was the right time to start making changes. There was never a day when I suddenly became less afraid of food, of gaining weight. All of these things came to me little by little, day by day, until without me even realising I was a different person. I was able to eat a sandwich without worrying about how many calories it had, I was able to pour out an extra five grams of oats by accident and not panic and pour them back into the packet. I was still an inpatient, but I was finding my freedom. I was finding my power.

Once again I decided to make a new rule around food: every time I saw a food and my brain told me I wasn't allowed to eat it, it went on my list of foods that I had to eat. At this stage in treatment I was allowed off the unit to go to shops and buy my own snacks, I was granted independence, I was trusted to take some responsibility for my recovery. I would spend so long wandering up and down the supermarket isles, wishing after the delicious foods that I hadn't eaten for so long, fantasising about myself buying and eating and enjoying all of the treats that were 'off limits' and 'banned', according to anorexia. So I turned it into a game – every time I left the store wishing I was 'allowed' to eat a certain food, wishing my eating disorder would be quiet for just a short while so I could buy something different, I made myself add the food to my list of snacks that I must try.

I built and built my list, waiting for the right time to start my challenges. But as with everything else, there was never a right time. There never came a day when I felt ready, so I just chose a day, and I did it.

It started with a caramel shortbread. It always used to be my favourite sweet treat before my eating disorder turned up – I would buy a pack of four decent sized pieces and they'd likely be gone in 24 hours or less. I couldn't resist them, but in the darkest days of my Anorexia I truly believed that I'd never enjoy one again. I felt absolutely terrified at the thought of bringing one back to the unit to have for evening snack – what would everyone think of me? Surely someone with 'real' anorexia wouldn't eat something as nice and indulgent as caramel shortbread, surely someone with 'real' anorexia wouldn't willingly bring back something that was so scary. And so came the ever-lingering thoughts of being a fraud. Of 'faking' my illness, of not really belonging in an inpatient unit. All of these beliefs flared up inside of me just because of one piece of caramel shortbread. But I powered through, and I headed out to buy my snack.

The first shop I went in, I looked at the calories on the packaging and freaked out so much I had to leave. Surely another shop would have a smaller piece, or one with less calories, so I set out on a mission to find a snack that was more acceptable to my eating disorder. I went into five shops. In all five shops the caramel shortbread looked exactly the same, they all had pretty much the same ingredients, and the energy content ranged by only 20 calories. Yet still I had a mission – a mission to find the caramel shortbread with the lowest possible number of calories. At that moment, the calorie count on a snack was the most important thing in my life.

The simple task of going out to the shop ending up lasting much longer than it should. And still I headed back to the unit with my shortbread, believing that this venture and the fact that I was facing one of my biggest fears, proved that I didn't really have anorexia. I ate my shortbread that evening, believing that this proved that I was cured of my eating disorder. I told myself I could see it in peoples' eyes – they knew that I wasn't ill anymore and they resented me for taking up a bed as an inpatient when other people were out there struggling to eat anything. While some people were out there, dangerously underweight and hitting rock bottom due to their illness, I was fine; I was eating caramel shortbread.

My head berated me for eating that snack, and all of the challenging snacks that came afterwards. But with each one I knew that I was recovering, and I knew that I was one step closer to beating the eating disorder. Looking back to the previous year, I never believed that I'd ever get to that stage. The stage where I was eating what I wanted, the stage where I could pick up a chocolate bar from the shop for my snack and have a tiny piece of me look forward to it.

As my time on the unit came to an end, I was challenging myself more than I ever had before. My list of foods to try became shorter as I was opening myself up to new experiences, new possibilities. I was still scared, but I worked through the fear. I still felt uncomfortable and guilty, but I fought through every negative feeling that anorexia threw at me in order to give myself the best chance at recovery. As I overcame more hurdles, the feeling that I no longer belonged on the unit grew. The last time I was discharged, I said that I felt like I'd outgrown the unit. But this time, I really think I had. My dreams and ambitions were too big to be held back by anorexia any longer, they were too big to be contained on an inpatient unit. This time I left with a smile on my face and my head held high – I was ready.

Dear Jade,

You're doing it. Everything that scares you, everything that makes your heart flutter and your hands shake. Everything you thought was too hard, everything you thought you could never do, you are doing it with unbelievable bravery and courage.

This is your time. This is your time to go forth and achieve everything you've ever wanted. After so long being held in chains, you are finally free.

Freedom isn't a path free of obstacles, it's the knowledge that you are strong enough to overcome all of the challenges you face.
Freedom isn't the absence of fear, it is knowing that you are brave and courageous enough to fight through it.
Freedom has no limits and knows no bounds. It is immeasurable. It is beautiful.

There'll be times when you still have to fight, and you'll feel like your own mind is dragging you down. But know that however heavy the burden feels, you can manage it; just like you've managed everything else.

Now you have found that tiny spark of freedom, you must hold onto it with both hands and never ever let it go. Don't let anything hold you down, because you deserve so much more than that. You deserve everything that this world has to offer. You deserve to

JADE KIDGER

fly.

HOLIDAY

The second time I was discharged from the inpatient unit, I was in a really good place. Although I knew that I still wasn't fully recovered, I felt more free, less restrained around food. I felt ready and motivated to maintain the weight that I'd gained during the admission. I was still absolutely terrified of putting more weight on, but I understood that in order to go back to university, in order to become a doctor, I would have to accept my heavier body. I had two months until the new semester began for my course and I was determined to get back. I was yet to be cleared by occupational health as fit to study, but they were the last hurdle I had to jump, they were the final barrier that stood in my way.

I can't pretend it wasn't stressful, waiting to hear what direction my life would be taking in two months time, but I did the important thing, and I managed to successfully maintain my weight.

I put all of my efforts into making the most convincing case possible for occupational health, and a month after I was discharged, a month before university started again, I got the news I was so hoping for. I was going back to medical school. I was repeatedly told that after fighting anorexia, getting through medical school would be a breeze – I could only hope that that would turn out to be true.

A couple of months after being discharged I felt like all of my dreams had come true – all the things that had kept me motivated throughout my admission were becoming realities, including a holiday in the seaside town that we'd been visiting my whole life. I don't think anyone can comprehend how much time I'd spent at the dining table, faced with my worst fears, pretending that I was relaxing on the beach and eating with my family. It was my safe haven, it was the place my mind would automatically go to when I couldn't stand my reality anymore. When I felt like giving up, when I felt like I didn't want to recover, I just thought about those amazing holidays and carried on with the knowledge that one day I'd be able to experience that again.

Although it was sooner than expected, although I didn't necessarily feel ready to challenge a holiday yet, I was so looking forward to the time away with my family, and unfortunately, anorexia. As far as I was concerned the illness was definitely not invited, but it was still intent on following me around wherever I went, and that included to the beach.

I was trying with all my might to hang on to that freedom that I'd discovered on the inpatient unit. I was constantly trying to build a wall against anorexia, but the foundations were slowly beginning to show cracks. The transition home had been positive, but keeping up the hard work was gruelling and demanding. Perhaps I'd let my guard down after I was told that I could go back to university. Perhaps I'd become too relaxed, too complacent when the battle was still ongoing. Whatever was going on in my mind, whatever wars I was still fighting, my strength and resilience were about to be tested greatly while I was away from home.

The eating disorder made its demands known before we left: no fish and chips around the harbour, no eating ice cream like everyone else, and no slacking on the exercise. Not that I was back to doing 'formal' exercise yet, but the brand new addition to our family, Ronnie the Labrador, made sure that I was regularly going for long walks and keeping my daily step-count up. How would I manage sitting down on the beach for hours at a time without keeping active? How would sitting still in a car all the way across the country affect my weight?

However much I wished to be left alone for just one week, the anxiety and the fear of gaining weight also joined us on holiday, and it made its presence known. Instead of sunbathing I would volunteer to walk the dog along the coast until we were both exhausted. Instead of relaxing I would take Ronnie out for exercise just to keep my steps up. When I was supposed to be getting dressed or going to bed, I would hurt myself as punishment for not doing enough, for eating too much, even though I was doing nothing different to normal.

On our first night away I sat on a bench overlooking the beach, and I felt so lucky to be alive. I felt blessed to have survived all of my fights with anorexia, and I felt hopeful that life could be good. And then my Dad turned up with paper packages full of fish and chips. Four meals – one for my Mum, one for my Dad, one for my sister, and one for my brother. And what did I do while they tucked in to their tea? I sat and wished more than anything I could be joining in with them. I sat while anorexia taunted me and teased me about eating my tea at home earlier, because I couldn't face having my favourite takeaway. I watched while my Mum tore off a bit of her fish to feed to Ronnie, and I wondered how my dog could eat more treats than I allowed myself to eat. Did I think he was greedy? No. Did I judge him for eating anything and everything people offered him? No. Did I think bad of him or love him any less because he ate ice cream every day, sometimes twice a day? Absolutely not. Why did I talk to my dog kinder than I talked to myself? Why did I love him unconditionally yet I still couldn't manage to love myself?

After sitting with the delicious smell of salt and vinegar wafting over to me and feeling insanely jealous, we went for a walk along the beach, and I was finally satisfied. The eating disorder was quiet for a bit, and I could enjoy the moment, knowing that while we laughed at the dog running in and out of the sea, enjoyed the sand between our toes, and appreciated the beautiful sunset, I was doing physical activity and burning calories. I was still catering to anorexia's every need.

During our mornings out doing activities – archery, mini golf, clay pigeon shooting, I would long for it to be lunchtime so that I could eat again. The thought of food never left my brain – it was a constant distraction, a continuous niggling at the back of my mind. At night when everyone else was eating ice cream and chocolate, I would feed the dog his ice cream so I felt like I wasn't missing out, while wishing more than anything that my mind would allow me to have an ice cream of my own. Despite the battles that I faced so far away from home, I did get chance to relax, and I did get chance to enjoy myself, but anorexia was always in the background, always waiting to strike.

Being away from home was hard: it was constant challenges, and it was feeling guilty for not allowing us to have a family meal out or get a takeaway together. It was attempting to enjoy myself while ignoring the screaming in my head, and it was worrying constantly about what I'd eaten and how much exercise I'd done. It was seven long, trying days that left me feeling worn out and exhausted, but despite all of these things, I had fun. I made memories, and I relaxed. All of the things my eating disorder had stolen from me and I'd worked so so hard to regain. Physically I was doing well – I wasn't gaining weight but I wasn't losing it either. I had more energy and I appeared much more outgoing that I'd been for a long time. I was due to regain the career that I'd had to put on hold and my future was looking good.

But the eating disorder still thrived inside of me. It still ruled my life in little ways every day, and it still forced me to constantly fight with myself. I wasn't yet a healthy weight for my body, but gaining any more was off the cards. I was no longer restricting calories to a specific number each day, but I still checked the energy levels of all of the foods I ate and anything I thought was too high in calories was banned. I'd stopped cutting out whole food groups from my diet but I was still placing restrictions on what I ate. On the outside it looked like I was recovering but on the inside I was still being held back. In many aspects I was better, I was finally eating again. I was doing well, but I still had my struggles. I still had battles to fight.

EXERCISE

I remember a time only a few years ago when I went to see my GP and she asked me how much exercise I did. I chuckled to myself and then admitted that I hardly did any exercise. I had a ten minute walk to and from school, I danced once a week, and I scraped through PE lessons doing the bare minimum. That was the extent of my physical activity. I know it's more than some people, but honestly, if I could have gone to school in the car I would have, if I could have gotten out of PE I would have jumped at the opportunity. I just simply didn't like exercise. I hated getting sweaty and out of breath, I hated feeling the burn in my legs, I hated everything about it. During the PE lessons where we were required to use the gym in our school, I used to sit on the rowing machine chatting to my friend, rowing exactly zero km for the whole hour.

I used to envy people who went to the gym every

day and went out running and kept really active. Just seeing them in their sports gear made me feel like I should be doing more. I looked up to them – they were doing everything that I felt too lazy and too sluggish to even attempt.

Bearing all of this in mind, when I decided to try and take up running in my second year of university I didn't meet a single person who wasn't shocked. 'Who? You? Running?' They would say. No one told me to my face that I wouldn't be able to do it, but I could see it in their expressions, hear it in their voices – no one believed that I'd ever really get anywhere. No one had faith that I'd stick with it, and if there's one thing I really love, it's proving everyone wrong.

So I began running. It was like nothing I'd ever known. It was like I was free. I'd finally found happiness in exercise and I relished it. I started small – a bit of running, a bit of walking, but after a few months I'd built up my stamina to allow me to run a few miles each morning. I felt so powerful and strong, I felt invincible. I'd get home, shower, eat my measly breakfast of fruit, and then go to my lectures, feeling drained and completely worn out but so smug and proud about what I'd achieved that morning.

Running became my release, my way to escape from the stress of medical school and studying. I would set out before the world had woken and it would just be me and the sunrise, burning bright in the crisp, clear morning.

On days that I'd been running I wouldn't allow myself to eat extra, even when my stomach was growling with hunger and I felt weak and shaky. I thought that the extra calories would cancel out the effects of the exercise. It's important to note that at this point, I didn't have an eating disorder. As far as I know my BMI was around the cut-off between healthy weight and underweight, but as I wasn't constantly keeping an eye on my weight, I can't be sure. What I would give to have that attitude again where I couldn't give a damn about what I weighed.

However reminiscing on these moments, I see the beginnings of anorexia lurking beneath the surface. I still hear my old housemate ask me if I'm eating enough, and I remember acting rather offended, but secretly feeling thrilled at the fact that I was obviously not eating as much as other people. I still see the exhilarating moment when I worked out my BMI for the first time in months and it was way below where it should have been, when I hadn't even been consciously trying to lose weight. It may not have been strong, and it may not have taken full control yet, but the eating disorder was being born.

Running might have started off as an innocent and wonderful hobby to help me feel fitter and improve my health, but before long it had become toxic. I carried on running into my third year, when the eating disorder raged through my body and mind, and the urges to exercise became stronger and stronger the more weight I lost. Suddenly, running wasn't fun anymore. I would start every weekend by going to my local park and doing a long and gruelling session, no matter the weather. I would brave the cold, the wind, and the rain just to stop anorexia shouting at me and telling me that it was unacceptable to stay in bed a moment longer than I had to. I would be forced to get up, bleary-eyed, and drag on my running gear, checking in the mirror that the tight-fitting leggings and top didn't show off my imperfections too much. I would leave the house foregoing breakfast and make my way to the park, often shivering and chattering my teeth due to the frostiness in the air.

Entering the park, and I would already be worn-out just from the walk, but that was no reason to give up and go home – I had a run to do. I set off and for about five minutes I was alright, it was manageable. But much longer and I was in agony. My chest felt like it would explode with the amount of air I was gasping in. My legs felt like they were detached from my body, carrying on moving of their own accord, because surely I wasn't strong enough to keep them moving myself.

In that moment my greatest wish was to stop. My greatest wish was to cease running and bring some feeling back into my legs, feel like I could breathe again, stop the ache and the burning surging through my calves. But I wasn't allowed to stop. All I knew in that moment was that if I didn't keep going the world would end. The illness was etching it onto my brain: 'just keep running, just keep running.' It became a rhythm, a chant, a champion's call. As long as I kept repeating those words I was okay; it took my mind off the torture I was inflicting upon myself, the abuse that I was putting my body through.

Every single time I finished what I'd set out to do. Every week it got harder as I had less and less energy, less and less reserve to keep me going, but anorexia wouldn't let me quit. It forced me to walk back home on shaking legs that were likely to give up any minute, it forced me to shower and look at my body after my run, and for once I was actually praised for my efforts – if I lay down my stomach wasn't just flat, it was concave. My pelvis stuck up into the air and for a minute the beast inside was happy. But only for a minute, because then it starved me until the afternoon. I'd just gone for a run – I couldn't ruin it by eating. The thought of food was crazy, any nutrition was off limits.

Anorexia made me treasure the feeling of faintness and weariness that it had worked so hard to bring me. It made me crave and long for that feeling with its twisted mind games and I brought right into it. I came to love that feeling, I came to cherish the shakiness of my legs and the twinges in my chest. I came to associate those feelings with hard work and achievement. I never saw them for what they were – warnings of a failing body, a body crying out for help.

Even after I was diagnosed with my eating disorder the longing for these feelings still persisted - exercise was part of my safety net, as long as I could exercise, everything would be alright. It made me feel ever so slightly better about eating and consuming calories. It made me feel like I'd achieved something, like I was worth something. Despite being warned of the danger that I was putting myself and my heart in by exercising, I didn't go very long without it.

I'm not too sure what drove me to disobey the doctors' orders and begin exercising during the early stages of recovery. I just know that one minute I was sat in my chair, bored, anxious, alone, and the next I was exercising in secret, breaking everyone's trust and ruining my recovery. And give anorexia an inch, and it will take a mile. I couldn't just stop after doing it once. It became an obsession, I was fixated on exercising as much as I possibly could. I hardly ever sat down when I was alone, and I didn't consider myself to be finished until my chest hurt. I would spend hours running around my home, running until I couldn't run anymore. It was just one more dirty little secret that my mind forced me to keep. Just one more way of isolating me and punishing me for starting recovery, for defying the eating disorder.

Months later, when I'd made so much progress and I'd been discharged from hospital, I still struggled with exercise. It wasn't intense, extreme exercise like I'd been used to, but still every step and every staircase that I climbed mattered to me. I couldn't face a day where I was predominantly sitting down, so I would make myself walk for miles to work off some of the food that I'd eaten. If there was an option to sit and an option to stand, standing would win every time. If I had to choose between getting the bus or walking, there would be no competition – walking it was. I never thought these things were significant enough to worry about. I never realised that they were tiny ways that anorexia was still controlling me. It was hiding in the shadows, while still making its presence known.

However, through all of the mess and all of the suffering that I have endured, I have discovered the magic of running. Although it was once a very detrimental part of my eating disorder, it has also allowed me to discover a new method of stress-relief and an activity which I genuinely enjoyed at the start, when my body was healthy and happy. As a child I never would have imagined that I would exercise for fun, but I know that in the future, when I am ready, it will become a big part of my life. I look forward to being able to run again when I can say that I don't want to go one morning because of the weather, and when I can stop and allow myself to have a rest half way through, and I look forward to coming in after my run and eating a huge breakfast, because I know I need the extra calories after my workout. I look forward to not counting my steps and not making myself walk to places when there is a much easier option. I look forward to living without having the constant worry about how many calories I've burned. I look forward to a life where anorexia doesn't win.

'Everything was okay. The sun was just biding its time behind the clouds, waiting to welcome her home.'

GOING BACK TO
UNIVERSITY

nowing that I was going back to university brought purpose back to my days: instead of getting insanely bored watching daytime television, I was studying to become a doctor; instead of taking the dog on endless walks to keep me occupied, I was learning how to save lives. I was busy, I was putting pressure on myself, but finally, after so long, my days didn't revolve around food anymore.

The last time I tried to recover I felt like I was nothing without anorexia. I didn't have a life, I didn't have a personality without the illness; my whole persona revolved around being sick; but now I was a student doctor. I was the very person I'd wanted to be when I was younger, I was a person who people looked up to, who they trusted with the most exposing and vulnerable aspects of their life.

I had to be strong now. People would expect me to look after them when they couldn't look after themselves. People would expect me to hold their life in my hands and protect it with everything that I had. Nobody wants a doctor with such a low BMI that they are in constant danger of collapsing, nobody wants to let someone who'd skipped both breakfast and lunch stick a needle in their arm. I knew that nobody would want to be looked after by me when I couldn't even look after myself. But I wasn't any of those things anymore. I was powerful, I was confident, I was a force to be reckoned with.

I was about to take a huge leap and live by myself in hospital accommodation, taking complete responsibility for all of the food that I ate. I knew that anorexia would tell me that I could get away with not eating, I knew it would try and force me to skip meals, but I was determined not to listen. I was hopeful: I knew this could be the turning point for me – a time when I could flourish. Despite my nerves about going back on placement after the disaster it turned out to be last time, I was more excited than I'd been in months. I was ready for this, I was intent on making this a success.

My first day on the ward I walked in right on time, so confident and composed, and I had full faith in myself. I got involved, I saw patients, I did exactly what I was meant to do – I learnt how to look after people. So why did I feel so completely lost and useless? Why, a couple of hours after that initial positive entrance, could I be found sobbing my eyes out in the toilet, planning my exit from medical school. Why did I go home that evening and hurt myself so badly that I'd still get questions about what I'd done to myself months later?

I felt like a complete failure. I felt like I was the weakest person in the history of humanity. I couldn't even last one day on placement, how was I supposed to become a successful doctor and work day and night to treat and care for some of the most vulnerable people in society? I went to bed that night sure that I was going to quit in the morning. But the day after this happened, I made one of the best and bravest decisions of my life. I walked back onto the ward with my head held high, and I got stuck into another day. I put everything that had happened previously behind me and I managed to smile and laugh and relax. It wasn't perfect, I was still finding my feet, but it was better; and I couldn't have asked for anything more.

As the weeks went by, I was completely smashing

life. Placement was getting better day by day, I was starting to really enjoy being a student again, I loved the independence of living by myself, I was eating every meal even though the eating disorder was telling me not to, and I was loving life. I truly believed that I was recovered. I truly believed that I had overcome anorexia.

I was still terrified to eat many foods, but I was eating three good meals a day, so that meant I wasn't ill anymore. I still got severely distressed at the thought of gaining weight every single week, but my BMI was high enough to be back at university, so I was recovered. I still weighed my food, I still restricted my calories, I still refused to eat foods with unknown calories and eat out, but anorexia convinced me that because I was eating, because I wasn't severely underweight, because I was functioning perfectly well as a medical student, there was nothing wrong with me. It told me that I didn't have an eating disorder anymore, but the fact that the voice was still there, in my head, telling me these lies just proves that I was wrong. This was just another trick that anorexia made me believe and I hate that I didn't see through it. I hate that I became complacent and took my eye off the ball. The illness almost succeeded in destroying me again.

I still had to get weighed each week, and each week, no matter what I'd eaten, I expected to gain weight. Most of the time I was right. I hear other people fighting anorexia saying that they want to gain weight more than anything. I hear other people getting frustrated when they lose weight, but that's not me. Even after all this time I hate the thought of gaining weight and I have never stepped on those scales and felt proud of myself or good about myself when the number has gone up. I have never stepped on the scales and felt sad or disappointed when the number has gone down. I know this is what's keeping me trapped. I know this was my downfall when I restarted university.

My weight was pretty much staying stable, sometimes going up slightly, sometimes going down slightly, but those little changes didn't bother me too much. It was only when I unexpectedly lost a significant amount of weight that my brain went into overdrive and I lost control again. To this day I still don't know why it happened – I'd eaten the same as usual that week, I hadn't done any more exercise than usual, but sometimes our bodies can be unpredictable, and for someone with an eating disorder that can be worrying but it is perfectly normal and okay.

The problem wasn't that I lost weight – weight is always changing, the problem was my response to the weight loss. The problem was that I felt ecstatic and elated at the loss, or rather anorexia felt ecstatic and elated. I felt exhilaration like I hadn't felt for months, I felt the dangerous euphoria that anorexia filled my head with when it was happy with me. I listened when I was told by my psychiatrist that I needed to eat a bit more, I listened when I was told I needed to restore that weight, but the eating disorder was already creeping back in. It was already getting stronger and it was getting ready to take back control.

It was more subtle than it had been before, but I was again being controlled by the eating disorder. In the past it had made me lose as much weight as quickly as possible, but this time, as long as my weight was dropping, it was okay however much it was. I knew if I dropped below a certain BMI I would have to leave university again, and this number was always in my head, threatening me. I think this is what saved me. I think this is what helped me to retain some of the logical side of my brain.

I still ate regular balanced meals, I still ate carbohydrates, I still ate something resembling a normal diet, but perhaps this made it worse, perhaps this just increased my denial. I didn't realise at the time that I was succumbing to the illness again, and neither did anyone else around me. Anorexia managed to disguise itself pretty well this time around, and if it wasn't for my weight slowly slipping down, I would never have believed that I was ill once more.

With each week that I lost a little more weight, it became ten times harder to gain it again. 'Just one more week', I kept telling myself, 'just lose a tiny bit more'. But this is how you get trapped. This is how anorexia wins. People were saying I was struggling, but I didn't agree – I didn't feel hungry or weak or exhausted like I did when I was struggling before. People were saying that I was getting to a point where I'd have to give up on my placement and my course again, but I didn't agree – I knew I wouldn't let it get that far. But I did. Every week I told myself that this was the week that I'd get back on track, but every week I delayed it, and every week I crept closer and closer to that fateful BMI that would well and truly ruin my life's ambitions.

Eventually I reached an ultimatum. I was mere grams off losing my place at medical school, it was time to decide who was going to succeed. It was sink or swim, eat or be eaten (literally). I knew I had to be stronger than I'd ever been before. I knew I had to triumph where in the previous weeks I had not. I had to just close my eyes and trust in the process. I had to have blind faith that the universe knew what it was doing. So I took a risk - I decided to save myself once more, and I prayed that it would pay off.

ENDING THE STIGMA

One afternoon a week throughout my placement I had to sneak off to see my psychologist. I would tell people that I had a 'personal appointment', and luckily for me no one asked for any more details. But I always wonder what I would have said if they'd have asked: would I have told them the stark and revealing truth, or would I have fabricated an elaborate lie to avoid any awkwardness and judgement? It's hard to know how people are going to react when you tell them a deep and personal truth like your mental health struggles.

I like to think that I hide my illness pretty well, and I'd love to think that if I told everyone about it, they would be really understanding and supportive, however the general lack of awareness around eating disorders puts doubt in my mind that people would react in the way I'd like them too. Of course, I'm making the assumption that the other students and doctors around me are mentally well. I'm presuming that they aren't fighting their own battles that they're just as apprehensive as me to reveal.

It's sad that there's such stigma and shame around mental health, I wish I could stand up confidently and proudly and announce to the world what I've been through (which is kind of what I'm doing in this book), but just like many other people, I am afraid. I am afraid to be an outcast. I'm afraid to be different.

Different shouldn't be a negative thing, like it is often seen as, different should be celebrated and honoured, because the world would be so boring if everyone was the same. I know that I'm different to many people on my course because I've had time off, and I've suffered, and I've spent a long time in hospital. But those details just embellish my story. They make my journey longer, but often, longer journeys lead to greater destinations.

Everyone is different, and I'm pretty sure everyone has things that they're ashamed of and want to hide. And that's okay, we don't need to lay ourselves bare for all to see, but for me I don't want something as big and as life-altering as anorexia to go unsaid. I don't want the two years of my life that I dedicated to recovery to be wiped out and forgotten as if they never happened. Anorexia does not define me by any means, but it has helped shape me and it's hopefully made me a more understanding and empathetic doctor.

The war that I've been through, and am still going through, is a part of my life whether I want it to be or not. And one day I will shout it from the rooftops. I will sacrifice myself to allow others to be free, to allow others to recognise that there is no shame in being mentally ill. I will take the judgement, and the nasty comments and all of the people that don't understand, in the knowledge that it will allow others to own their eating disorder and be proud of everything that they've fought through.

MY NEW LIFE

Seven days after I made the choice to save myself, I was back to be weighed. I knew that I was about to find out whether my medical career was still viable or whether I'd let the best opportunity of my life slip down the drain. I could see as soon as I walked in that my psychologist was set up to deliver bad news, I knew that she believed that I would once again have lost weight. But I knew different - I could feel it in myself that I'd gained weight this week.

I stepped up to the scales feeling confident yet apprehensive. I knew I needed to gain weight, I knew I *had* gained weight, but deep down inside I knew that I still wasn't ready. I kept telling myself that weight gain was good, weight gain was liberating me from my eating disorder, but as much as I wanted weight gain this week to allow me to stay at university, another part of me was disappointed in myself.

The eating disorder was screaming at me for 'giving up' at the pivotal moment. It was telling me that it would have been better to have to leave university again – it would mean I was sicker, it would allow the illness to stay with me longer, it would bring me approval and acceptance from my mind. But why would I want any of that? I was starting to become tired of the games and the hurt. I wanted to defeat it properly this time.

I stood on the scales and the number went up, just like I knew it would. It went up just enough to take away the threat of me leaving university, and I accepted it. I wasn't happy about it, it didn't feel good, or like I'd achieved anything amazing, but I accepted it nonetheless. I realised that although this was progress, I was still so far from being fully recovered. Despite living away from home and still eating, despite being deemed 'fit to study' and being allowed back to university, I was still ill. I had allowed myself to eat more over the week but I was still restricting by choosing the food with the least calories, by not eating when I felt like it, by not eating what I really wanted. I had gained weight, but it was the absolute minimum amount that I needed to gain to stay at university. It was hard to admit, but my life was still being micromanaged by the eating disorder and I needed to find a way to break free.

I knew this wasn't the recovery that I wanted,

I knew that I didn't want to spend my whole life avoiding big, juicy burgers, and greasy fish and chips, and huge family-size sharing blocks of chocolate just because a pathetic little voice in my head told me I didn't deserve them. I was slowly coming to terms with not being critically underweight and so ill I could barely function, but just like I wasn't living my life back then, I still wasn't living my life now. I was eating, but I still couldn't go out for meals to celebrate my families' birthdays. I had a good balanced diet, but I still couldn't go to the cinema and share a bag of sweets with my friend. I ate foods that I liked and that I wanted, but I still couldn't snack throughout the day because I was hungry, or pick up a spontaneous takeaway when I couldn't be bothered to cook, or accept a cupcake or a piece of chocolate off someone just because they were being kind. That's the life I wanted, not this life stuck in limbo half way between illness and recovery, where I was still being haunted by anorexia, even if it wasn't trying so hard to kill me anymore. I knew that if I was going to do this properly, I had to commit completely. I had to eat whatever, and whenever I wanted. I had to be valiant and daring. I had to be my own hero.

It started that afternoon. I made a promise to myself, a promise to eat whatever I wanted. A promise to stop counting calories. I promised to satisfy my cravings and properly fuel my body. I promised myself that while I didn't have to like the weight gain that was going to come, I was going to accept it and move on. I knew it would be hard, I knew it would be scary, I knew it would be painful. But I also knew that this was the only way that I was going to beat my eating disorder once and for all. There was no way around it, there were no shortcuts or tricks to make it easier. I knew that I was going to be putting myself through a whole different kind of hell than what I'd already been through, but most importantly of all, I knew it would be worth it.

I went shopping, and I bought all of the ingredients for my new life. It took an awfully long time agonising over what to get and building up the courage to buy foods I feared; but eventually my first task was complete. One small step for Jade, but one great leap in the quest to destroy anorexia. It gave me so much anxiety, putting all of my shopping away, knowing that at some point I was actually going to have to eat it, but I knew that this was just a small taste of the anxiety that was going to befall me on my great journey to complete freedom. I went into my bedroom and I tore up my meal plan. I found planning extraordinarily helpful when I was first in recovery, but now it was placing limits on me – I didn't want to be bound by the decisions I made on a whim at the beginning of the week, I wanted to be spontaneous, I wanted to eat whatever I fancied in the moment. I felt hopeful, I felt motivated.

A few hours later I went into the kitchen to make my evening meal. It took what seemed like forever to decide what to have; I had the whole world available to me, no foods were off limits now. And in the end I chose porridge and toast. It may not seem like a particularly big fear food, especially when I could have chosen a whole pizza or a huge plate of pasta or a massive portion of cheesy chips, but for me it was a win. I was eating 'breakfast food' at six o clock in the evening. I didn't work out exactly how many calories were in my meal, but I knew it was more than usual. I was eating both porridge and toast, a combination I'd been scared of eating since being an inpatient because it felt too indulgent. I sat down, I ate everything without a second thought, and it was delicious. My journey had truly begun.

The following day I woke up and the guilt hit me. What had I done yesterday? The panic overtook me, the only thought running through my mind: 'I have to restrict, I have to make up for how greedy I was yesterday'. I couldn't believe I'd been so stupid, why did I think it was a good idea to let go and recover from my eating disorder? But wait a second, isn't recovery what I wanted? Isn't that my ultimate goal, to be free of this constant onslaught of hate by the cruel and vicious voice in my head?

In the past I would have simply skipped breakfast and moved on, maybe even felt proud of myself, or strong or powerful. But I'd made a promise to myself, the most important promise I had ever made. So I sat myself down and I thought logically – one day I wanted to wake up and be able to eat whatever I wanted for breakfast without feeling bad or guilty about it. The only way that would happen is if I got rid of anorexia, and the only way to do that is to do the opposite of what it says. So I chose to do what scared me the most, and I ate my breakfast.

Recovery doesn't just happen, I knew that I wouldn't simply wake up one day and be free of my demons; I had to work for it. I had to be dedicated, and every time it made me feel awful about myself, I had to fight through the feelings with courage. The urge to look at calories was incredibly strong. No matter what the food was, no matter whether I'd had it a million times before, I still found myself searching the packet for the nutritional content every time I contemplated eating or buying something. I don't quite know when I thought they'd changed the calorie content of strawberries, I'm not sure why I expected the bread that I bought every week to suddenly have twice the number of calories in it, but checking made me feel at ease, it made me feel safe. I know I told myself I wouldn't count calories anymore, I know I promised myself that I'd stop, but it terrified me. Sometimes I would do it automatically, I would catch myself and be momentarily angry, but then relieved that I had the information that I so eagerly sought. I thought that I had to stop myself eating too much, but I soon came to realise that there was no such thing as 'too much'. Food is fuel, food is energy. Our bodies are insanely clever at processing the energy we give it, I knew that I had to learn to trust mine, I had to have confidence in myself.

After that first week of aiming for freedom, I put on the largest amount of weight that I had ever done in one week. All I wanted to do was curl up into a ball and shut myself off from the world. I was asked how I was feeling, what I was thinking but I couldn't put it into words: there were emotions flowing through my head but they were all jumbled up into one big mass of negativity. It was like nails on a chalkboard, or a buzzing in your ear: I knew that it was bad, and I knew that I wanted it to go away more than anything, but I couldn't quite describe how it felt.

Everything was too immense to process – my fear and my discomfort were too huge to contain in one body, anorexia's outrage and fury too loud and too intense to allow any other thoughts in. But after I was weighed, I stumbled outside into the sunlight, breathed a breath of fresh air, and something wonderful happened: I let it go. All of that feeling, all of that emotion that was too big to contain; I watched it flutter away into the big wide world and get lost in the beautiful afternoon sunshine. It tried its damn hardest to fight its way back to me but I wouldn't let it touch me anymore: I was winning. I was going to enjoy the glorious day and eat every single crumb of my lunch on the luscious grass, and feel happy to be alive. The eating disorder was not invited.

Dear Jade,

This is the first day of the rest of your life without anorexia. Everything will feel wrong, you will feel fat, greedy, weak, a failure. But that is the eating disorder talking, and it is NOT your friend. It will tell you to stay with it just a bit longer, it will try to convince you that you are nothing without it. But that's not true – without it you are free.

You'll never feel ready to recover, because anorexia doesn't want you to recover. It wants to kill you. I know recovery is scary, but being stuck with anorexia for the rest of your life is absolutely terrifying.

Do it to become a doctor. Do it to eat fish and chips at the seaside. Do it to eat cheese whenever you want. Do it so you can go out for meals. Do it for chocolate. Do it for everyone who loves you. Do it for yourself.

It doesn't have to be perfect. There will be good days, bad days, easy days, and hard days. You just have to be strong. You have to get up everyday to fight the same demons that left you so tired the night before. That is bravery. Bravery is not missing lunch or skipping breakfast. Bravery is hearing the voice and being strong enough to defy it. Bravery is listening to your body and allowing yourself to eat. Bravery is holding on for one more day when all you want to do is give up. I know you're so tired, but you CAN do this. Don't be too hard on yourself, and more importantly, believe in yourself. You are capable of

JADE KIDGER

amazing things.

MY BODY

I've always had an up and down relationship with my body. When I was a child I remember being called 'fat' by a girl in my class when we were getting changed for P.E. I remember wearing a bra before everyone else that I knew and being incredibly self-conscious about it. I remember struggling to get changed for swimming in front of people without showing off my tummy or my chest or my legs. When I was just twelve years old I remember eating a brownie at a birthday party while the birthday girl's aunt chanted 'a moment on the lips, a lifetime on the hips'. Like many other little girls, I saw pictures of celebrities in magazines and wondered what was wrong with me – why wasn't my tummy flat? Why weren't my ribs showing through my T-shirt? My memories of my body as a child are clouded by anxiety and concern over how I looked.

I occasionally look back on pictures from when I was a child and I don't see any of what 8 year old Jade thought she looked like. At the time I would have probably described myself as 'chubby' and 'plump', and looking back perhaps I would have been right. But what wasn't right at the time was the negativity I associated with my body. Yes, I was a bit bigger than some of my friends, and maybe I had a tiny extra bit of fat around my middle, but I also had a bigger personality, and a tiny extra bit of sparkle in my eyes.

I could run around the playground, screaming with joy and not run out of energy after a few minutes. I could sit and write stories for hours and hours without having to take a break because my concentration was waning. I could talk and talk and talk (just ask my parents) about anything and everything, because I wasn't too exhausted to hold a conversation. I never appreciated how lucky I was to be in a healthy body. I never appreciated all of the things that the body I didn't particularly like allowed me to do and enjoy every day.

Growing up I became much more educated about the non-realistic body types that were displayed by people in magazines, and I was proud to not compare myself to these people anymore. I came to understand that it wasn't normal or healthy for someone's ribs to be showing through their t-shirt. I was taught that having a more rounded tummy, or a bigger chest, or broader shoulders was beautiful. But still I was seeing other peoples' bodies and wondering why mine was so different, wondering why my body was so ugly when everyone else's was perfect.

I don't think I've ever seen a person and thought that their body was not beautiful. In the height of my eating disorder my mind managed to convince me that I was a bad person, that I thought anyone who had a big tummy or a round face or thick thighs was unattractive and imperfect. How else would it make sense for me to be so scared of attaining these things if I didn't see them as negative qualities? I thought that if I was so terrified of gaining weight myself, I must hate and look down on everyone who was heavier than me. I thought that if I found it unacceptable for myself to become bigger, it must also be unacceptable for anyone else to be bigger than me.

Through all of the confusion about my thoughts and feelings, and my body and food at the time, I thought that this was one thing that made sense. It played on my mind until I was absolutely disgusted with myself. What right did I have to determine whether someone else's body looked nice or not? What right did I have to judge anyone?

I began to look at people walking down the street. I began to look at all of the differences between their bodies which were at a healthy weight, compared to my emaciated body. I began to imagine what I would look like if I put weight on. Here's the funny thing – every single body that I saw, whether they were a healthy weight or whether they were overweight or underweight, looked beautiful.

What surprised me even more was that when I began to imagine whether that person was good or bad, kind and caring or selfish and mean, I wasn't looking at their waist size or their clothes size, I was looking at their smile. I was watching how they treated people around them, and I was looking to see whether their eyes lit up and their faces radiated positivity and warmth. I realised that those qualities were so much more important to me than how much somebody ate or how much they weighed, so why didn't I believe the same for myself? Why was I still utterly convinced that people would be judging me on my weight and my eating habits, rather than my personality and warmth, which I'd just proven to myself were much more important?

All around me I saw people accepting their imperfections and owning their body. I saw people posting pictures on social media with their bloated tummies and stretch marks and I was jealous. I was in absolute awe of anyone who could love and respect their body enough to want to inspire others. I looked up to people that embraced their individuality and had enough courage to shout about it to the world. I wished so much that I was able to love myself. I wanted more than anything to look at my tummy in the mirror and not hate what I saw. I tried, I really tried. I kept repeating the same things to myself: 'I am beautiful', 'I am strong', 'I don't have to be skinny to be loved', but however hard I tried, I still couldn't accept my body. I looked at myself every night and I hated the way that I looked.

I felt separate from my body – I felt like it was betraying me by making me so self-conscious and miserable. I would take off my clothes and step into the shower, and every time I looked down I despised what I saw. As much as I desperately wanted to change my thoughts around my figure, it's not as easy as just forming a different opinion and sticking to it. I couldn't force myself to love something that I didn't, I couldn't make myself accept something which to me, was unacceptable.

I would always read inspirational quotes about loving your body, and throughout my recovery I read so many things about how to accept weight gain and how to be more body positive; but the more of these things I read, the more

I was convinced I was broken. I knew gaining weight meant gaining my life back, I knew it meant that I could go back to medical school and become a doctor, but I couldn't stop wishing for a smaller body. I couldn't stop detesting what was happening to me, what I was doing to myself. Until one day when I'd been in recovery and having these feelings about myself for two years.

I was tired, I was weary, and I was exhausted. In case you've never experienced it, hating yourself is hard work. I wanted nothing more than to just curl up tight and recruit the safety of my bed to make me feel vaguely human again. But I didn't do that, instead I looked in the mirror. I stood in the same position for what must have been at least half an hour and just stared at myself. Started at my body. My body which I took to the brink of death, but which managed to cling on to life to give me another chance, even when I was convinced I didn't want one. My body which always seemed to put the scariest amount of weight on, even when I cried at it and cursed at it, because it knew that that's what I needed to be healthy. My body which allowed me to get into medical school. My body which allowed me to make amazing memories. My body which gave me energy to move and dance around my bedroom and do absolutely anything I ask of it. It never once betrayed me, it betrayed anorexia. My body was on my side this whole time, even when I felt like it was plotting against me. My body saved my life. My body, the strong and unbeatable warrior.

FALLING IN
LOVE

After so long trapped in the darkest recesses of my mind, I can finally see a way out. It may seem far away, and it may feel hard to reach, but freedom will wait for me. It doesn't matter if I take baby steps or great big leaps, I WILL reach that escape.

After so long hating my body, hating what recovery has been doing to it, I can finally say that I've fallen in love. I've fallen in love with myself. I've fallen in love with my big, bloated tummy, and my round, chubby cheeks. I've fallen in love with the muscles in my legs that no longer protest against any form of exercise. We're fighting as one now. Just me and my body against the world.

I know this next phase will be hard, but I don't care anymore. Throw everything at me – misery and hate, I will acknowledge it and move on, knowing that these feelings are only temporary. Every time anorexia tells me that I can't do something, I'm going to prove it wrong and succeed. I'm going to kick its ass and show it who's boss.

I hope that in the future I'll look back on this time and be proud of myself for how hard I've worked. I hope future me will recognise all of the effort I've put in to give her a life, and I hope that she'll take nothing for granted. I hope that she'll love her life and do what really makes her heart sing, and more than anything, I really hope she'll eat the chocolate bar and not give a damn what anyone says about her. I hope she'll be truly happy.

'*With every step she took, with every moment she left behind, she started to become whole again.*'

COMING UP
FOR AIR

My body was changing and I was scared. What I was eating was changing and I was scared. My weight was changing and I was scared. But recovery is scary – as the nurses on the inpatient unit used to tell me: 'if it's not scary, you're not doing it right'. And while I don't believe there's a single 'right' way to recover from an eating disorder, I do know that the way that I was trying to recover for so long was wrong. I now know that allowing myself to eat more but still restricting my calories wasn't proper recovery. I know that giving myself more energy but exercising to compensate wasn't proper recovery. I know that by staying completely in my comfort zone and not taking risks, I wasn't properly recovering. To finally be rid of the eating disorder, to finally be free from the restraints that it placed over me, I just had to bite the bullet and eat.

Despite my worries about my weight and my body, I felt liberated and free. Every time I chose to eat something with more calories in it I felt the anxiety rage through my mind, but I knew I would survive. I knew that anorexia was becoming weaker, and I was beginning to triumph over it at last. I could go to the supermarket and not be limited to just a couple of sections. I could buy new foods that were higher in calories because I was no longer trying to restrict myself. I could eat what I wanted, because the eating disorder was no longer in charge. I'd opened up a whole new world of options – peanut butter sandwiches, chocolate milkshakes, creamy, cheesy pasta. And that was just the start. My determination grew stronger, and my longing to be truly free dominated the thoughts in my mind. I could still hear the eating disorder, I could still feel its rage, but I knew that I could overcome it. I could overcome anything.

I was battling through the discomfort, and I was fighting the voice every step of the way. I was gaining more weight each week, and although it was painfully hard, I didn't give up. Sometimes I stood proud with my head held high, and sometimes I was hanging in there with only my fingertips. But the important thing is, I never surrendered. I remember a time when the thought of gaining this much weight would have sent me spiralling into a major breakdown. I remember a time when I thought that if I ever gained this much weight I simply wouldn't survive. I thought that the world would stop turning, I thought that life wouldn't go on. But every week I was overcoming more challenges than I ever thought I could endure. I was conquering my demons. I was becoming a soldier.

Everything was going well. I was in control, I was making the decisions now. I told myself that every decision I made around food, I would stop and think: 'Is this what anorexia wants me to do or what I want to do? Which decision will take me further away from my eating disorder?' Every choice was a conflict between anorexia and life, the illness and Jade, suffering and freedom. It wasn't hard to know what the right option was, but actually doing the right thing was unimaginably tough. The 'right thing' ranged from having a little bit more cucumber with my tea, to having an extra snack mid-afternoon simply because anorexia was telling me that I couldn't. Everything that it said I couldn't do I did with more drive and more motivation than ever before. I wanted to beat this. No one was forcing me to eat, I was doing it all on my own. For the first time in my recovery, I was the boss.

Everything changed one afternoon, when I couldn't stop thinking about the cereal bars in my fridge. When my mind was so preoccupied with food I couldn't think straight, I listened to anorexia tell me that there's no way I could have a cereal bar, I listened to it tell me that it wasn't the right time to eat, and then I went to the fridge and got my cereal bar. I was shaking, I could barely breathe, but I ate the snack and I ignored the voice shrieking inside my head. I felt like I'd done something naughty, I felt like I'd done something bad, but somewhere inside me I knew I'd done the right thing, the brave thing.

All I could think in that moment, was now that I'd worked up the courage to eat a cereal bar, I could do anything. There were no rules now, my body was crying out for food and even though I was terrified of what was happening, I was terrified of myself and terrified of my body, I went against all of my instincts and I ate another cereal bar. And once I started I couldn't stop. It felt like coming up for air after being under water for so long. I'd starved my body of what it needed, so when I was finally able to take a breath, I breathed until I could breathe no more. The body craves that which will allow it to heal and survive - it didn't matter what the food was or how it tasted, to my body it only mattered that it was food, and that it would deliver the calories that I'd deprived myself of for so long.

I ate until my fridge was empty but my belly was full. I ate even though my stomach hurt and I felt like I would burst. I ate anything and everything I could find, almost on autopilot. I couldn't control my body, I couldn't control myself. It's like I was in a trance, and when I couldn't take a single mouthful more, I woke up. I woke up and I was devastated. There were no words to describe the shame, to describe the embarrassment running through my head. I was absolutely mortified. Instantly I wanted to take back what I'd done. I would have paid any price to be able to click my fingers and go back in time. 'Why were you so weak? Why did you give in to the temptation so easily?' anorexia yelled. It was more furious than ever before, and this time I couldn't ignore it: the screaming was too loud.

I felt immense horror and incommunicable fear. My first thought was about my weight, my second thought was about the number of calories I'd just consumed, and my third thought was about how greedy and disgusting I was, how revolting and repellent people would find me if they knew what I'd just done. I thought I'd failed at having anorexia, I thought I'd failed at recovery. Barely a month into my commitment to rid myself of the devil, I'd somehow gone spectacularly wrong. I wanted to hide under my blanket and never ever come out. I wanted to fall asleep and never have to wake up. I was convinced I would never get over this, I was convinced that this was the end. The end of me, the end of the world, the end of life.

I didn't know what else to do, so I did the only thing I could think of in my panic and terror – I made myself sick. I made myself sick non-stop for two hours, and afterwards I still felt dreadful. My panic was receding but a new emotion was beginning to brew – anger. I was so mad at myself. I was mad at the world. But mostly I was mad at anorexia. How dare the illness do this to me? How dare it make me feel this useless and distressed? I'd sworn that I wasn't going to let it win, yet here it was battering me and abusing me with its vile and nasty insults. It was more vicious than ever before and I couldn't cope with its attacks any longer. My body was exhausted, my mind was exhausted, I was ready to give in and succumb to the voice. But I managed to find one last tiny spark of power, and I promised myself that I would try again tomorrow.

But tomorrow eventually came and the events of the previous evening were still careering around my head. It was impossible to think straight, and I was so bloated I'm sure people would see my huge tummy underneath my clothes. Although the previous night I wanted to turn back time and erase what had happened, now I wanted to fast forward until I could forget. Until I could feel the blissful ignorance of not remembering what I went through, what the voice put me through. I swore I wouldn't eat that next day, I swore I'd punish myself for my gluttony and self-indulgence. I knew it was anorexia who was telling me to punish myself, I knew the eating disorder was the one shouting and screaming in my mind until it was impossible to ignore, but I couldn't fight anymore. I was weak, hadn't I proved that by binge-eating? So I resorted to what I knew best – starving myself.

As time went on the torment eased and I dared to eat again. I was so scared of losing control, I was petrified of bingeing again, but I overcame my angst to push forward in recovery. I tried to get back to where I'd left off, but I was more cautious and more hesitant now that my worst fear had been realised. I had to learn to trust myself again, to have faith in my body again. Nobody knew about my slip, it was my skeleton in the closet, my biggest sin that would disgrace me if it ever got out. But I managed to pull through. I managed to survive something that I thought would be the end of me. Until it happened again. And again and again and again...

MY DOUBLE
LIFE

My eating disorder once again made me believe that I had recovered, that I was okay. It made me think that it was dying, that it was becoming weaker and weaker every day. I thought that if I was bingeing and 'allowing myself' to eat that much food I couldn't possibly have anorexia anymore. If I could deal with consuming that many calories, I couldn't really be ill. But I wasn't dealing with it, I wasn't dealing with it at all. I had unlocked a new method of torture, a new version of the devil who was stronger and more persistent than before.

My double life had begun. By day I was a strong capable medical student rushing around the wards, assisting other doctors, taking part in surgery, but by night I was breaking. While my fellow students went home and studied for our upcoming exam, I went home after not eating all day, and wreaked complete havoc on my life. I would binge, and afterwards spend hours forcing myself to vomit, on multiple occasions I vomited so forcefully that I lost control of my bladder. I would hurt myself, I would unleash all of my frustration and all of my anger upon myself in the form of horrific violence and brutality. I would sob until I had no more tears left to cry, until I was too exhausted to even have a shower.

I would crawl underneath my blanket and wish for salvation. I would pray for sleep to come so that I didn't have to hurt anymore. But I never won – the sooner I fell asleep the sooner the following morning would appear. Then I would have to drag myself to the wards and pretend all day that there was nothing wrong. But I knew that when I finally found relief from the lies and the deception at the end of the working day, I would have to go through hell all over again.

I had thought that being an inpatient and surviving my darkest days was the hardest thing I'd ever do. I hoped I would never have to face anything comparable to that ever again, but I was wrong; being in hospital wasn't the hardest thing I'd ever done. This was. Pretending I was fine when behind closed doors I was the complete opposite of fine. Sitting with my eating disorder in the early hours of the morning, alone and frightened, and listening to it confirming my deepest and darkest fears. Fighting against myself all of the time but having to hide any sign of weakness, any sign of fragility from everyone around me.

I was so tired I could barely carry on. Every morning it was a horrendous struggle to get out of bed, to take my tablets, to get dressed, yet still I pushed myself to my absolute limits. I worked my mind and my body to exhaustion to keep up the façade that there was nothing wrong, when more than anything I wanted to give up.

Each time I binged I would burn my wrists as punishment. In the moment I didn't care what damage I was causing, I didn't care that it was agony, or that it was dangerous – it was the only way I could express my hurt. It was the ultimate punishment for this 'crime' that I was addicted to committing, and then when morning came I would have to think of a way to cover it up so I could still lead this double life. I would shake with the pain, but it was the only thing that kept me going. I believed at that moment in time, that it was my only option, that I wouldn't survive the anxiety and the hurt without the scars and the weeping wounds on my arms.

Every day I promised myself that it would be

the last time I did it. Every day I swore I would make a change, but every day became harder and harder as I was drawn further into the depths of this new-found anguish. For me this was new territory, it was a galaxy that was undiscovered. I was used to not eating enough, I was used to starvation, but suddenly my life had completely turned on its head. I'd been thrown head-first into a war which I was completely unprepared for.

Instead of feeling empty and constantly battling my intense feelings of hunger, I was uncomfortably full and left wishing I felt hungrier at meal times. Instead of being weak and frail I was stronger and heavier than ever before. But I still wasn't happy, I was still struggling, regardless of my weight. Before I thought that restriction and binge-eating sat on opposite ends of the spectrum, but now I know that they fight from the same side. They both left me feeling guilty and anxious about my body and weight and food. They both left me mentally exhausted and they both made me just want to curl up in bed and sob. They're both ways of coping with life. They're both methods of projecting my worries and anxieties onto food. They're both nasty, disgusting bullies whose main aim is to see me fail.

I thought because I was gaining weight I was getting healthier, but I couldn't have been more wrong. Just like I used to lie in bed feeling my heart beat slowly and wondering if I'd survive the night, I once again found myself in the same situation, but my heart was fast this time, rapid and strong. Was it beating that way because of all the vomiting? Was I at risk of having my heart suddenly stop like all of the literature says it might? Just like before when it was almost too much effort to speak, I once again saved my words, but this time because of the severe pain that invaded in my throat from being sick so much. While before I was rarely warm enough to be without a hot water bottle, now I was having hot flushes and sweats, my body was turning the extra energy I'd given it into heat. I no longer looked ill, people didn't stare at me anymore and wonder what was wrong with me, but looks can be deceiving. I was still very much in the clutches of my eating disorder. I was still trapped. I was still desperately searching for an escape.

Each night I sat alone in my room. There was nothing and nobody that could distract me from my distress. Whereas before I was surrounded by people, whether it be my family while I was at home or the staff while I was an inpatient, there was no one that could save me now. The only voice I could hear was that of anorexia, the only thing I could feel was its hate and spite. I was a solo warrior, no army behind me, nobody to convince me to fight when I wanted to surrender. Of course my family were still supporting me from 50 miles away, of course I still saw my outpatient team once a week, but who was there to hold me and comfort me in the middle of the night when the voice was deafening? Who was there to look into my eyes and tell me everything was going to be okay in my deepest, darkest moments? I felt more alone than ever. I felt weak, I felt fragile, I felt pathetic. The littlest thing was enough to set me off. Every day I was sinking further and further into the abyss, and every day it was becoming harder to survive. I was being torn apart by my own mind.

I knew that I was rapidly gaining weight: I could feel my tummy getting bigger by the day; I could feel my clothes getting tighter and tighter, even the ones I wore before I became ill. My belly felt enormous; I no longer had a flat stomach, even first thing in the morning when I hadn't had anything to eat or drink. Whereas losing weight felt familiar and commendable, this weight gain felt horribly unwelcome and unsettling. The shame that I felt before about my eating, when I was trapped in the depths of anorexia, was nothing compared to this – this was too huge to comprehend. This was too powerful to fight against. I became more terrified of stepping on the scales than ever before - I dreaded seeing what

I'd done to my body, I dreaded anyone else seeing what I'd done to myself. For a month I refused to be weighed. For a month I wouldn't let anyone see the consequences of my bingeing because I was so ashamed.

But the longer it went on, the more I realised that there was absolutely nothing to be ashamed of. I may have felt like I was eating too much food, but there is no such thing, especially not in anorexia recovery. My body was in dire need of all the calories, all the energy it could get its hands on. Some people say that there is no such thing as a binge in recovery, they call it extreme hunger. But to me it didn't matter what it was called, whether it was binge eating or extreme hunger – it was the scariest thing I'd ever experienced in my life. It was torture, it was agony, but deep down inside I knew that I was giving my body what it craved, what it so desperately needed.

BURNS

As my first placement back at medical school drew to a close, I was really struggling. My days were constant cycles of restrict, binge, then self-harm, and every night I'd lie in bed feeling hopeless and defeated. Every night I'd lie in bed regretting skipping breakfast the day before, regretting giving up too easily when the urges to binge consumed me, regretting torturing myself at a time when I should have shown myself forgiveness and compassion. I would sit in the dark with the overwhelming sense of despair threatening to consume me, and I would cry. I would cry for that young girl who never deserved any of this pain. I would cry for the broken soul who at the start of recovery was so optimistic. I would cry for the past version of myself, the version that would eat a whole pizza and enjoy it, walk down the confectionary isle of the supermarket without panicking, who would enjoy a sausage sandwich without experiencing a paralysing fear of putting on weight.

One evening alone in my room, I spent hours burning myself late into the night. I would withstand the pain and agony of one burn, just for anorexia to tell me that my efforts were pathetic, that to properly show my torment I would have to inflict much more damage. Every time I tried to stop and go to bed, my mind would drag me back up and force me to carry on, to continue the torture that I was unleashing upon myself. I wasn't allowed to run my arms under cold water, I wasn't allowed to put cream on the wounds to ease the discomfort, I wasn't allowed to take any painkillers: the voice told me that I deserved this pain, that it was payment for disobeying it. Over the next few weeks I would have to wrap my arms in clingfilm whenever I wanted to wash my hair to stop the warm water and shampoo running into the open wounds. I would have to endure the soreness of my clothes rubbing against the raw areas of skin and the itchiness of the healing scabs.

I knew that I was giving in to the eating disorder, but I couldn't stop. I wasn't allowed to stop. Part way through this long and tortuous episode my phone began to vibrate, and out of curiosity I paused the punishment for long enough to read the message that I'd been sent. It was from my

Mum - nothing special, just saying goodnight, but I began to think. How ridiculous that I was loved this much, yet I still felt the need to subject myself to this abuse. How ridiculous that I am lucky enough to have people in this world to live for, to recover for, yet I'm determined to continue sabotaging myself.

A few days later I went home in order to prepare and study for my upcoming exam. I couldn't hide the burns, I couldn't pretend that I was coping when I so clearly wasn't, but I was terrified of putting my family through the immense stress and worry of seeing me suffer. Nevertheless, I divulged to them what had been happening, what I'd been experiencing during my time away, and it turned out that the more I divulged, the lighter my burden became. It didn't take away the hopelessness that sat with me every night, or the despair I felt when I was sure I would never recover from this illness, but just for a moment, I shared my load. Just for a moment, I let myself be reassured and comforted and told that everything would be okay.

Dear Jade,

You are very nearly there. You've come so far, you just have to hang on for a tiny bit longer. Right now it feels like the pain and the distress will never end, but I promise you that it will. You WILL be happy again, you WILL find peace.

You've struggled with this for two years now. That's two whole years of your life that've been taken away from you. You do not deserve this, you deserve to have a beautiful life full of freedom and laughter. I know you're exhausted, and I know you're ready to give up, but you have to be stronger now than you've ever been before.

I know that you lie in bed at night and doubt that you'll ever recover, but you CAN recover, it is possible, you have to believe in yourself. I know that you sit and wonder whether you'll be stuck like this for the rest of your life, but this won't be forever, because you are a warrior, and I know that you will never stop fighting.

When the hard times come, remember that you are loved and that you are safe. When your mind is torturing you, remember that whatever it's saying is wrong and that it won't always be like this. And when you feel like giving up, remember that you are strong, you are capable, and you are brave.

Have faith in yourself. You can do this.

SCARS

There's rarely a battle that doesn't leave scars. The wounds and the pain endured during a fight are almost bound to leave their mark, whether physically or mentally.

The scars from my battle sit proudly upon my body. Once something I was ashamed of, they now tell the story of my journey, of my hard and harrowing journey. They show that I never gave up. They show that however hard life got, whatever was thrown at me, I hung in there. They represent a story of hope, a story of survival. They represent the story of a brave, courageous soldier. For so long people have asked about my scars and I've refrained from telling them the truth. I tell them that I had an accident in the kitchen, or I fell and grazed myself. But I finally feel ready to tell the truth. I finally feel ready to stand up and own my story and my scars. I'm not scared anymore – if people don't understand, it's my job to educate them. If people ask me to cover up, it's my job to show them that no one should have to hide their scars. I'm not ashamed anymore. I'm ready to open up to the world. I'm ready for the world to hear my story.

'Her resilience was breathtaking,
her determination magnificent.
Courage shone out of her, filled her
very core. She was more beautiful
than she could ever imagine.
She was more extraordinary
than she would ever know.'

PROGRESS

Admitting to my psychologist that I was having trouble binge eating was exceptionally difficult. I wondered whether she would be as disgusted with me as I was. I wondered whether she would think I was a horrible person. I wondered whether I was her first ever patient to do this – to go straight from severely restricting my intake to eating huge amounts of food in just a couple of weeks. Even saying the word 'binge' made me feel sick, it made me want to run away as fast as humanly possible; anything to stop myself hearing that word, that word which I feared so much.

But in the end I managed to swallow my pride and admit what had been happening behind closed doors. I admitted to the agony I was putting myself through, the terror that I felt each and every night when I went to bed. I couldn't look at her while I was saying it, I couldn't stand to see her reaction. This felt like the biggest revelation of my life, it was ten times harder than telling people I had an eating disorder in the first place. But once again, just like every other time that I'd spilled my secrets, my words were met with understanding and reassurance, comfort and caring.

We agreed to work on my problem together. We agreed that the reason for my binges was not eating enough, not eating regularly, not nourishing myself like I should have been doing. We agreed that I would gradually build up to eating three proper meals and three snacks every day. I was terrified – I knew that amount of food would make me gain weight, yet I also knew that when I restricted it led to a binge, which made me put on weight anyway. In that moment I would have done anything to stop the binge-restrict cycle, I would have done anything to escape the pain and mental torture that were constantly befalling me. I knew this chance was my lifeboat, and I couldn't let myself drown any more.

I was ready to make changes. I was willing to listen, to learn. If it would take away the horrendous guilt and self-loathing associated with bingeing, I was ready for anything. Over the next few weeks I increased my food intake. I began to add in snacks in a bid to fuel myself adequately so that my body was nourished, and

I began to eat bigger meals that were properly balanced so that my body got everything it needed. It was an enormous challenge, it was overwhelming at times, but after weeks of trying, after weeks of fighting, I finally managed it. For one whole week I beat my eating disorder at every turn. I fought through the bloating, the feelings of fullness, the feelings of guilt and greed, and I ate. I ate my lunch when I was still full from my morning snack. I ate my snacks even when I didn't feel remotely hungry. I showed my body love, and I showed it the compassion that it so deserved.

I ate caramel shortbread for the first time since I challenged it as an inpatient. I even ate it stood up on a train – an insignificant achievement for many, but a huge achievement for me. And that very same day, the same day that I had to buy a new coat because my old one was too tight across the chest, the same day I had to buy trousers with a waist two sizes bigger than usual, I challenged one of my biggest fears - I ate a cheeseburger from McDonalds. I could have chosen just a plain burger. I could have chosen something with less calories, in fact that's what my head was screaming at me to do. But I knew that I'd been craving that cheeseburger for months. I knew that for months I'd been denying myself that burger because I was simply too fearful, too afraid of the consequences. I can't tell you where my courage came from that day, I can't tell you where I suddenly managed to cook up that amount of bravery, but I can tell you that I was proud. Yes, I felt anxious and guilty and horrible, but I was proud.

A few days later I walked into my next session with my psychologist. I walked in with dread and trepidation, I walked in with unease filling my mind. Despite making incredible progress, despite winning so many battles and overcoming so many hurdles, there was still something that frightened me more than anything else, which sent shivers of terror running down my spine – getting weighed. I thought that I'd be used to it by this point in recovery, I thought that I'd have found some magic solution to relieve me of the crippling anxiety, to absolve me of the soul-destroying distress that befell me when I was asked to step on the scales, but I'd had no such luck.

I knew that I couldn't avoid being weighed any longer, I knew that despite the fact that I'd gone a whole week without bingeing, despite the fact that I'd had so many moments over the last week to be proud about, seeing my weight was going to be agony.

With my whole body shaking, with my knees

knocking together, I stepped up to the scales. I didn't dwell on what was about to happen, I didn't even think about it. I just stepped on and looked the number that appeared. The number which was bigger than any I'd seen on that display before.

I'd hit my target BMI. In fact, I'd exceeded my target BMI. This was the most I had ever weighed. This was the highest BMI I'd ever had. A universe of feelings erupted in my mind – panic, fear, disappointment, shame, helplessness, revolt, and most surprisingly, grief. I grieved for my emaciated body with a ridiculously low BMI. I grieved for my empty stomach and my bones sticking into my mattress. I grieved for the burning in my legs and the ache in my arms when I had next to no muscle. I grieved for the comfort and sense of achievement the eating disorder brought me.

I'd spent so long expressing my mental pain through my body, through physical means, and now they contradicted. My body was healing but my mind was just as addled as ever. My body was becoming whole but my mind was still broken into tiny pieces, impossible to fit together. But despite my healthy weight, despite no longer meeting the criteria for a diagnosis of anorexia nervosa, I knew without a doubt that I wasn't yet recovered. I'd come so far on my back-breaking, exhausting journey; but I knew that I still had so far to go.

For the first time in an appointment, I spent the whole hour attempting to stop the tears streaming down my cheeks. Once again I had to bear hearing the two words that felt like a knife stabbing its way through my heart: 'well done'. I had to endure the screaming of anorexia and its vile words and threats – threats forbidding me from ever eating that much food again. Threats telling me that if I was to put any more weight on I would be punished. I would be punished in ways worse than I'd ever been before. I left that appointment in a state of total panic, in a state of overbearing anxiety.

The following week saw me slipping back into my old ways. I once again turned to my deadly comfort blanket for when things felt too big and too scary to handle. I fell back into the same methods of restriction that I'd used time and time before, and just like I'd proven in the past, that led to more binges. I wish I could have held on for just one more week, just one more weigh-in. Maybe I would have gained some confidence in my body, learnt to trust myself.

But that one week full of victories taught me that I could do it. I was strong enough, powerful enough to overcome anorexia. Although I returned to old habits, I was still battling; I was still working each and every day to overcome everything that was thrown at me. I may have taken a step backwards, but it was merely one step back, compared to the hundreds that I'd taken in the right direction.

Although I knew that there were hard times on the horizon, I also saw the possibility of there being better times, times when I could live a somewhat normal life, a somewhat happy life. I continued to fight, and although each week was excruciatingly difficult and there were many times that I slipped up, I always managed to push through. Despite my struggles, I was hopeful. I was hopeful for the future. My life wasn't perfect – far from it, but I felt more stable than I had been for a long time. Although I still struggled, the voice wasn't as strong, it wasn't as dominant. Every day, I was making small, but very real steps towards recovery.

To Anorexia,

I never thought that I'd be writing to you two years on. I never thought that you'd still be a part of my life. I thought, and hoped, that you'd be long gone, a distant memory, a figure left in the past.

But we won't dwell on what could have been. I want to focus on the here and now. Despite all of your efforts, I am still here. Each and every obstacle that you've put in my way, I've overcome them. It hasn't always been easy, I'll give you that. You've tried your best to break me, and sometimes you have succeeded, but I will always find a way to put myself together again.

You can break my heart, but it will continue to beat. You can break my mind, but it will continue to fight. You can break my soul, but it will continue to live.

I am brave, and I am loved. Two things that you'll never experience, two things that you attempted to tear away from me. But they are in my blood. Bravery and love run through my veins, and they exist and thrive in every single cell of my body. They are the very core of my being.

Each and every morning, as the sun rises, you rise alongside it. When I wake up I can feel your presence – haunting me, stalking me. Yet still each night I rest easy, knowing that one day I will wake up and you will be gone. Driven out by my courage and determination. One day you will cease to exist. I will have beaten you, and I will finally be able to find peace.

MY CHRISTMAS WISH

Despite the eating disorder staying very much alive, I achieved a lot over the next few months. I passed my medical school exam, something which a couple of years ago I never thought I'd get the opportunity to sit, let alone pass. I completed my next placement at a primary school, getting stuck in even on days where I didn't think I could get out of bed. My birthday came around and for the third year in a row I didn't manage to have cake, but I did manage to have pizza with extra chorizo (my absolute favourite)! I worked up the courage to buy a chocolate advent calendar, and finally, on the 12th day of December, I was brave enough to open the first door.

Some weeks anorexia dominated my mind. It

would ruin me until I thought I had nothing left to give, but I always managed to find a tiny glimmer of hope. I would manage to pull myself together again for a while, only to once again fall apart a couple of weeks later. It was still so hard and still so painful, but gradually the tough weeks started to become less and less. The sunshine would stay for a little longer and the dark clouds became that tiny bit easier to push away.

I still struggled with both food restriction and binge eating, but some days I managed to eat 'normally', I nourished myself properly, and on those days I felt such immense pride. I learnt to sit with the anxiety and guilt until it began to ebb away, and I learnt the importance of putting the previous day behind me and focussing on the future. Things weren't perfect - I still struggled, I still cried, I still felt like giving up, but ever so slowly, my power and my strength were returning.

As Christmas came ever closer, I found myself contemplating the future. I would look up at the beautiful twinkling lights and feel that childish hope and optimism that next year would be different, that next year would be magical. I could have asked the universe to grant me joy, I could have prayed to the Gods to grant me happiness, but deep down inside I knew that there was only one person that could make my Christmas wishes come true. There was only one person who could fix me, only one person who could save me, and she was one of the strongest and bravest people I'd ever known. She was a hero.

Although I kept reminding myself that it was just another day on the calendar, and that I shouldn't put too much pressure on myself, I was looking forward to Christmas. The first one in three years where I could at least attempt some of the delicious dinner that my brother made. I was looking forward to a Christmas without a hospital admission looming in the near future. I was looking forward to a Christmas where I didn't stare longingly at the chocolates, where I didn't load my plate with salad but wish more than ever that I was eating stuffing and pigs in blankets. My anxiety was high, but I was more determined than ever to conquer my demons. I knew it was only one day, but I also knew that there hadn't been a single day in a very long time when I didn't still carry anorexia with me, when I didn't still have to fight. I was continuing on the long, winding road to recovery, but I wanted more than anything to make this Christmas special, to make this Christmas the first of many happy ones to come.

I still had so much healing to do leading up to the holidays. I still had to struggle through each and every day, despite everyone else being merry and bright. Just because everyone else was happy, it didn't mean my illness disappeared. Just because people were wearing silly festive jumpers and novelty musical ties, it didn't mean fighting my eating disorder was any easier.

A few days before Christmas I was looking back at last year's photo that we took in front of the tree, and I wished that I was in that place again. That place where my clothes were hanging off me, where my body was smaller and more fragile. I thought back to this time last year and I remember eating turkey salad while everyone else ate their Christmas dinner. I remember trying to play a board game but not being able to concentrate on what was happening. Despite these things I longed for my broken and skeletal body; I yearned for that feeling of sitting down and having my bones protrude into the chair, that feeling of hunger which I know plagued me throughout the day. But I was more determined than ever not to let the eating disorder triumph this year. I was determined to battle through Christmas with every last fibre of strength I could find within myself.

I knew that when I sat down to dinner with my family, my hand would be shaking when I put the stuffing on my plate. I knew that if I managed to eat dessert I would have to try and distract myself from the guilt for the rest of the day, but I also knew that these little victories would be worth it in the end. I knew that each and every step forwards I took, the closer to recovery I was getting. Christmas day wasn't going to be easy – far from it. But I knew that I would be surrounded by my family, and I knew that whatever happened, whatever anorexia put me through that day, I would be safe and I would be loved, just like I was each and every day.

Dear Jade,

I know that you're still struggling, and every day is agonisingly hard, but I want you to know that I'm proud of you. In those moments when you've wanted nothing more than to crawl under your blanket and never come out, I'm proud that you decided to resurface. In those moments when you've cried into the middle of night, I'm proud that you woke up the next morning and tried again. In those moments when you've slipped up or had a setback, I'm proud that you managed to put it behind you and get back on track.

I'm proud that during the toughest battle of your life, you stand up each and every day with courage and dignity, all while facing the huge challenges of being a student doctor in a global pandemic. I am proud that you choose to continue your life when the illness is trying so hard not to let you. I'm proud that you are still fighting two years on, even though you never imagined it would be this tough.

You are so much stronger than you think – you have endured so much more than you were ever prepared for, and despite being continually knocked down you have never failed to get back up again. I'm proud of every single scar on your body and every single molecule of your being. I'm so immensely proud of the journey that you've been on, and all of the mountains that you have climbed, and storms that you have faced. I can't describe how it feels, looking back over everything that you've done over the past couple of years – you have proven to everyone that you can withstand anything that life throws at you. But more importantly than that, I hope you have proved to yourself how incredibly courageous and resilient you are. I hope you have learnt to love yourself.

It doesn't matter if the future is uncertain – what matters is that you are here right now. On this very day. Surviving and breathing. Living. Life is beautiful. Laughing is beautiful. Love is beautiful. YOU are beautiful. Know that you are infinitely loved and appreciated, and you make the world a better place by simply existing. Know that you are strong and capable of spectacular things, and you are admired for all your efforts. Know that you are enough just as you are, and you don't need to be anyone else.

I know it's hard, I know you're exhausted, and I know you feel like you have nothing left to give. But you WILL be okay. You WILL get to see the light on the other side of this storm. Just keep fighting with every ounce of your being, I have complete faith in you. You just have to start believing in yourself. Hope and happiness can always be found, even on the darkest day, even when your mind is intent on torturing you with malice. The darkness never stays. The sun will always rise again.

So whoever you decide to be, wherever you decide to go, embrace life. Be thankful for the good, and be accepting of the bad. Be loving, be kind, and be proud. Be proud of yourself in every way that you can, and don't ever give up, because one day you will set yourself free.

25TH
DECEMBER 2021

I've made it to Christmas day, 2021.

I woke up this morning weighing the most I've ever weighed. It's scary, it's uncomfortable, it's anxiety-provoking; but it's also what I need to live. To properly live, free from any restraints, free from anything holding me back. However this year I've woken up with so much more than that: I've woken up with a strong and healthy body that will let me take Ronnie the dog for a Christmas morning walk; and I've woken up with a tiny glimmer of hope, a tiny spark of courage that I pray will last for Christmases to come, that I pray will carry me through all of the battles I have yet to fight.

Today I've had tears streaming down my face, and for once they were tears of laughter, not tears of distress. I have eaten pigs in blankets, I have eaten stuffing, and I have embraced every challenge and every opportunity that has come my way. At times I've felt anxious, I have felt like I wouldn't make it through the next minute or the next hour, but when my anxiety feels too big to contain, too strong to handle, I feel safe with the knowledge that it will pass, just like every other time that I have felt like this.

Despite the struggles that I've faced throughout today, I can't remember the last time I was this happy. I'm tired from fighting, tired from battling through my anxiety, but for once I am at peace. Although the voice is still within me, although I know I have many more battles to endure, for once I am content. I know that I'll more than likely wake up tomorrow and feel the fear all over again, but right now, in this very moment, looking out at the dusk falling on this beautiful Christmas day, I am hopeful for a future without the eating disorder. I am hopeful for a good life in which I am free.

For over two years now I've been sure that this suffering will never end, that this phase of my life will never come to a conclusion, but I now have faith that one day it will. Maybe not today, maybe not tomorrow, but I see a future with freedom, a future with joy and happiness. I know that anorexia will continue to try its best to break me for however long I dare to survive. I know that it'll always be with me, lingering in the shadows, but I also know that I am stronger than the eating disorder. I know that I will never, ever give up the fight because I have amazing things to live for. I have love and hope and bravery – things that anorexia will never have.

At the minute my life has a lot of ups and downs – one week I'll win and the next anorexia will make the score even. The monster fights on, but I fight harder. It sometimes wins, but my victories are bigger, bolder, braver. Throughout my journey there have been times when I thought I wouldn't survive, there have been times when I didn't want to survive. I have seen and done things that I never thought I would have to experience, but every single hardship that I've fought to overcome has been worth it to get to today.

I am not giving up. I will never give up because I know that somewhere out there is the life that I dream of. The life that I'm meant to live. There are times when I'm not locked in battle, and I'm smiling. The times when I'm not being broken down, I am totally, unequivocally whole. Each night I go to bed and I close my eyes, thankful that I am still here. Thankful that I held on when it seemed impossible. Thankful that I had enough resilience and strength to fight back when it seemed the world was against me.

My future looks bright – I'm on course to become a doctor; I have a healthy and happy family who will continue to support me through thick and thin; I have the drive and determination to beat anorexia, I just have to accept that it will take time, and I must remember to forgive myself when I make mistakes. I feel strong enough now, I feel brave enough. I know that whatever next year has in store for me, I will get through it with grace and dignity. Every day I will strive to make myself proud, even if it's just by rolling out of bed and brushing my hair. But I will also strive to show myself compassion in the moments that I don't feel proud of myself.

Whenever I'm going through a hard time I like to look up at the night sky and believe that everybody's destiny is written in the stars. I like to believe that the universe has a plan for each and every one of us, and that for me, in the right place, at the right time, everything that I've been trying to achieve will happen. And with immense courage and incredible determination from me we will make it work; I will be free of anorexia for good.

My journey has been long and rocky. Every hill has felt like a mountain, every rain shower has felt like a thunderstorm. But I know that along the way I have learnt so much about myself and about life. In two weeks I will begin my placement in psychiatry as a medical student, and I am determined to use my experiences to make me a better doctor, a more understanding doctor. There are many times when I wish I'd never had to embark on this journey, but I know that without it, I wouldn't be as confident, as caring, and as strong as I am now. Through the bruises and the hurt I have somehow evolved into something unstoppable, something fearless. Today, and every day going forward, I am a warrior. I will fight until the very end, and one day, I will be free of everything holding me down. I will finally be me again.

*'And just like that, she knew.
She knew with all of her heart
that it was her time to go forth.
To conquer everything that was
trying its best to hold her back.'*

To anyone who is struggling,

Please, please keep fighting. I know that it's tremendously hard, and I know that there are times when you feel like this will never end, but after the storm there is always light. Although the sun sets every evening, there is always a dawn.

If you were waiting for the universe to give you a sign, to tell you to keep going, to tell you that you do not deserve to suffer, this is it. This is me telling you that on this day, and on every single day yet to come, you do not deserve to be in pain. You deserve so much more than the distress and the agony that your mind is putting you through. You deserve all the love and care in the world.

I promise that there is a way through the torture, through the torment, and there is hope and freedom and happiness waiting out there especially for you. I know that you may feel like the only way forward is to suffer, but just hold on a tiny but longer. Hang in there with everything you have, because the pain that you're feeling right now, it won't last.

You are so loved, and you are needed in this world, even though your mind may be telling you otherwise. Your mind may be telling you that you're worthless, that you don't deserve to be happy, but know that you deserve every single ounce of happiness on this planet. You are more than worthy of a beautiful life, a life full of love and laughter. A life where you can be whoever you want to be with nothing holding you back.

You are perfect. Every little thing about you is perfect. Every flaw, every imperfection that you believe you have, they are beyond beautiful. And you are stronger than you could ever imagine. You are more resilient than words can say, and you have so much bravery within you, it oozes from every pore. You may not feel like it, but you are incredible. You are still here, living and breathing, and that in itself is a magnificent achievement.

I can't give you a reason why you're going through this, I really wish I could. I wish more than anything that I could hold you tight until you feel safe, and tell you that everything will be okay, that you will be okay. I wish that I could save you from the agony, shield you from the pain. I wish that I could make all of your suffering disappear, I wish that you didn't have to go through any of this.

But we can't change the past, we can't take away the pain and the terror that you've already had to endure. However we can change the future. We can fight to make a wonderful life, a life where we are not held in chains. We can battle to be free, free of every single thing that is currently holding us down. Although you may not be able to see your army fighting behind you, although you may feel incredibly lonely, know that you are never, ever alone. Never forget how extraordinary you are, you brave and fearless warrior.

Lots of love,
Jade xxx

ONE FINAL NOTE

When I was younger I wanted to be an author more than anything, but I always thought it too hard, too unrealistic. So I am beyond excited to finally fulfil one of my greatest wishes, even if it has come after a long and terrible period of suffering. I can't tell you how many dreams I've had about writing this book, how many times I've lain in bed thinking about holding the finished product in my hands, how many times I've woken up in the early hours of the morning with ideas that make me have to instantly get up and write them down so I don't forget. I'm going to say something now that I haven't been able to say honestly for years: I am so damn proud of myself. Not just for surviving anorexia, but for writing everything down and sharing it with the world. But I'm not just proud of myself, I'm proud and eternally thankful to some other people too:

My Mum – for staying strong when I was growing ever weaker. For understanding what was going on in my head, even when I couldn't understand it myself. For loving me unconditionally even when I didn't smile, and my illness made me a horrible person to be around.

My Dad – for forgiving me when anorexia expressed its anger through me; it was only so angry because you cared so much. For driving a three hour round trip just to keep me company for an hour, outside in the freezing cold when I was an inpatient during Covid. For always believing in me, even when I was hopeless and I didn't have any belief in myself.

My sister – for stepping up to your big sister duties brilliantly when I needed someone to be there for me. For giving up your bed so willingly so that I could have our shared bedroom to myself, so that you wouldn't give me a cold when I would have been too weak to fight it off. For taking me out to the cinema when I was barely allowed to leave the house – those films became the highlight of my week.

My brother – for always offering to help me out should I ever need it when I was in hospital.

For keeping my car shiny and clean even when I wasn't allowed to drive it. For always being kind and funny, even in the dark times.

And of course, thank you to my wonderful dog. I never thought I would meet such a sweet, loving dog; I love you so much. You always know when I need cuddles and support. You deserve all the sausages in the world for being a truly amazing friend.

Behind every soldier there is an army. Behind every victory there is a battle. There are so many more people who helped me on my journey and helped me to get my life back. In fact there are too many to name, but you know who you are. Having an eating disorder is one of the hardest things in the world, but watching someone that you love suffer and battle for their life, sometimes that's even harder. In my weakest times, I have been shown strength. In my darkest times, I have been shown light. In the times when I was so close to giving up, I have been shown resilience and determination.

However many times it may have felt like it, this has never been a solo fight. I hope everybody out there struggling knows that they never have to fight alone - there will always be someone who wants to help, who will lend a shoulder to cry on. One of the bravest things you can do is reach out for support, and I hope that after reading this book, you realise that getting help isn't a sign of weakness, it's a sign of the utmost strength and courage.

This is not the end...

...this is just the beginning.

Useful Numbers and Websites

Beat Eating Disorders (England):
Call: 0808 801 0677
Email: help@beateatingdisorders.org.uk
Website: www.beateatingdisorders.org.uk

Mind:
Call: 0300 123 3393
Website: www.mind.org.uk

Samaritans:
Call: 116 123
Email: jo@samaritans.org
Write: Freepost SAMARITANS LETTERS
Website: www.samaritans.org

YoungMinds:
Text: YM to 85258
Website: www.youngminds.org.uk

About The Author

Jade Kidger is currently a medical student in the UK but loves writing in her spare time. She writes about her struggles with mental health and things that helped her through the tough times.

When she's not studying or writing, she loves reading crime thrillers and taking her beautiful Labrador for walks in the Derbyshire countryside.

Jade would like to say a huge thank you to everyone who reads (and hopefully enjoys) her books - she is forever grateful.

Printed in Great Britain
by Amazon